July 17

Con ▓▓▓▓▓ ə Disease

What Patient Stories Teach Us

Karen P. Yerges
and
Rita L. Stanley, Ph.D.

Foreword by
Lesley Ann Fein, M.D., MPH

Seeking Help by
Robynn Harris

Copyright © 2005
by
Karen P. Yerges and Rita L. Stanley, Ph.D.

The information contained in this book is for educational
purposes only.
Discuss your healthcare concerns with an appropriate
medical professional.

ISBN 1-4196-2165-3

LCCN 2005910572

The Mitre's Touch Gallery
1414 Adams Avenue
La Grande, Oregon, 97850
United States of America

(541) 963-3477
www.confrontinglyme.com

To my daughter, Tess,
a child patient, who won
her battle with Lyme disease.

Karen P. Yerges

To my husband, Dr. James C. Stanley.

Rita L. Stanley, Ph.D.

Acknowledgments

The authors, Karen P. Yerges and Rita L. Stanley, Ph.D., would like to thank all of the Lyme disease patients and their families who volunteered to be profiled in this book.

Lauren
Glenroy Wolfsen
Danette MacDonald Cade and husband, Charlie
Nancy Oace
Linda Rinaldi and family
Michael and Rebecca Daniels
Sue Ferguson
Christie and Greg Smith
Lynda McDonnell
Miguel Perez-Lizano and Bo
Joan and Kevin McComas
Michelle and Kevin O'Leary and children
Rhonda
Edwin Lilley

We would also like to thank Dr. James C. Stanley and Adrianna Stanley for providing technical support, encouragement, and advice; and David L. Yerges for his editorial direction and production management.

The following persons are also acknowledged for providing encouragement, guidance, reviewing and information for this project: Dolly Curtis, Heather Gadberry, CMT, Joel M. Shmukler, Esq., Karen Vanderhoof-Forschner, Pam Weintraub, and Jim Wilson.

Cover Design

We would like to acknowledge and thank David L. Yerges for designing the cover with its visualization of Borrelia burgdorferi spirochetes under high magnification.

Foreword

We would like to thank Dr. Lesley Ann Fein for her constructive review of our manuscript and for contributing a powerfully insightful foreword to this book. She has been a tireless advocate for the health and welfare of Lyme patients, not only as a dedicated physician, but by serving as the Medical Director for the Lyme Disease Society, and as an advisor to the Lyme Disease Foundation.

Seeking Help

We are especially grateful to Robynn Harris for her written contribution to this book, Seeking Help. A Lyme patient and founder of numerous support groups, Robynn offered some of her best advice for patients seeking diagnosis and treatment for Lyme disease and other tick-borne illnesses. We're honored to have her contribution in our book.

Contents

Foreword

When I was asked to write the foreword for this book, I had conflicting emotions. Should I try to discuss only the scientific debate, or should I present what I believe to be a wider, deeper, and more complex aspect of the Lyme disease controversy? It became clear to me that the global perspective must be discussed to more fully understand the depth of emotions surrounding this complex and greatly debated disease.

I became interested in Lyme disease in 1982, when the first cases were being presented at Mt. Sinai Hospital in New York City, where I did my internal medicine residency. This was the first infectious disease which had clearly been shown to trigger autoimmune disorders. The concept of autoimmunity, however, would seem to be counterintuitive to those who subscribe to the theory of evolution. Why would an organism allow for its body to reject parts of itself as if they were foreign invaders?

It was then that the study of Lyme disease became fascinating to me. I attended the first conference on this disorder in 1984 and began to read whatever material became available on the subject. After moving to New Jersey and establishing a private practice in 1988, I started looking deeper into cases of lupus, chronic fatigue, fibromyalgia, and arthritis and wondered if some of them really exhibited the long-term manifestations of Lyme disease. Some patients clearly had Lyme disease, others did not, and some patients seemed to fall somewhere in between. Over the years, I presented my findings at the annual international conferences hosted by the Lyme Disease Foundation. In 2003, I co-chaired a conference with Dr. Brian Fallon, Professor of Clinical

Psychiatry, Columbia University College of Physicians and Surgeons.

In the early 1990's, as a physician who diagnosed and treated many Lyme disease patients, I became a target of investigation by insurance companies. This did not sit well with me since I knew that many of the sickest patients responded very slowly to treatment and often required far more treatment than insurance companies were allowing.

The situation became very contentious in 1993 through 1995 when I was asked to sit on a panel of experts discussing criteria for the diagnosis and treatment of Lyme disease intended for use by insurance companies. There were heated debates. I was one of the physicians vocally opposed to establishing overly restrictive criteria which would be used by insurance companies to deny coverage. When the majority leader of the New Jersey Senate at that time, saw the level of disagreement, he invited a group of us to meet with him to discuss legislation. The intent of the legislation was to mandate insurance coverage for at least 12 weeks of intravenous antibiotics as treatment for Lyme disease. It came as a shock that not only did we have opposition from specific academics, but also, from radical patient groups who opposed the concept of any limits to therapy. We tried twice to get this legislation passed but failed both times to get it through both the Senate and the Assembly.

Interestingly, the Lyme vaccine trials were beginning at about this time, and the CDC surveillance criteria were being discussed. The definitive criteria for the diagnosis of Lyme disease resulted directly from the need to objectively define the disease in order to perform the vaccine studies. How could you decide if a vaccine is preventing a disease, if you have no accurate definition of the disease itself?

Thus began a dark era where patient welfare took a backseat to more market-driven concerns. Test kits were patented based upon specific strains of Lyme bacteria which were designed to differentiate vaccine recipients from natural cases. While this approach was useful for vaccine testing purposes, it was not appropriate to use these kits and these criteria to screen the general population for Lyme disease. To this day, the current CDC criteria do not include tests for the most common antigenic variants seen in the general population. Before the human clinical vaccine trials, we also knew that animal studies suggested possible adverse reactions to the product if there was existing infection, and human studies had confirmed that Lyme could trigger autoimmune disease in genetically predisposed individuals. How then could anyone conduct studies on the general population without screening for these risk factors?

Around the same time, the researchers conducting these studies were solicited by insurance companies to write guidelines for the diagnosis and treatment of Lyme disease. These guidelines imposed stringent restrictions on diagnosis and treatment and ensured that many patients being treated for Lyme disease would not be covered by their insurance companies. Concurrently, physicians who utilized the knowledge they gained from attending conferences and reading the wealth of studies from both the United States and Europe, realized that this illness could become chronic and progressive. They understood that some patients would need months to years of treatment before a successful clinical outcome was ensured. The perspectives of these physicians were clearly at odds with the dogma perpetuated by insurance companies. Many of these insurance company experts lectured at academic medical centers and presented the position that those who treat Lyme disease as a chronic illness were "quacks" and "mavericks" and should be put out of business.

I was one of the many physicians put in the uncomfortable position of deciding whether we should follow our hearts, our clinical judgment, and the Hippocratic

Oath or to play it safe. Should we insist on treating this disease as aggressively as possible to avoid the devastating consequences of permanent arthritis, multiple sclerosis, and a host of other sequelae of incomplete treatment? Or should we play it safe and follow the artificially devised, restrictive guidelines, and avoid inquiries, investigations, and complaints by insurance companies and state medical boards?

It is not in my nature to allow anything to compromise my ethics, so I chose the tougher route. I have faced harassment by insurance companies, threats by local hospitals, and threats to revoke my license, but I am firmly convinced that I am doing the right thing. I have seen Lyme disease transform brilliant minds into confusion, dementia, and profound depression. I have seen athletes develop crippling pain, weakness, and confinement to wheelchairs. I have also seen that with enough treatment, nutritional therapy, and exercise regimens, these same people can return to normal.

This is not a debate about the science. This is a brutal attack launched by a few influential physicians who have aligned themselves with insurance and pharmaceutical companies against individuals who threaten to expose the underlying misconceptions and deceptions and who have the courage to continue to treat patients correctly despite threats and intimidation tactics.

This book represents patients who are seen on a daily basis by physicians, like myself, who treat Lyme disease. Physicians, who courageously treat these incredibly sick patients, deserve the highest respect from the medical profession rather than the condescending and scathing criticism to which they are subjected almost daily. There is a silver lining: a growing group of legislators and lawmakers, who are recognizing this injustice and forging the way for change.

I want to thank the authors for this moving and brilliantly written book, and I am honored that they have chosen me to write this foreword. I would also urge all those physicians who are treating this disease to continue to fight for your patients because the tide is turning.

Lesley Ann Fein, M.D., MPH
West Caldwell, New Jersey
September 2005

Introduction

"There is only one cardinal rule: one must always listen to
the patient."
—*Dr. Oliver Sachs, British neurologist*

What is it like to experience a chronic
illness? The experience is truly difficult
to comprehend for those who have never
been personally affected. Try to remember how it felt—
mentally and physically—when you were sick or suffering
from an injury. Then imagine having no idea when or even
if your pain and debility will end. Perhaps you will get better
for a while only to relapse again and again. Your prognosis
is unknown, and while you cling tenaciously to hope, there
is every chance that things might get much worse.

As a result, you may become dependent on caregivers
who are as unsure as you are of your situation. You have no
idea about what will happen to your job, your family, or your
finances. Since no one is affected more than you by your
illness, the burden of discovering a knowledgeable physician
lies squarely on you. Following a strong survival instinct, you
search for answers—the causes and treatment options—and
you must do all of this discovery while possibly suffering
with disabling symptoms. You try to explain your situation
to those in close contact, not to invite pity, but acceptance,
respect, and most importantly, loving support.

No one is ever really prepared for serious illness
when it happens. Dealing with the physical and mental pain
and the associated losses can only be learned by living the
harsh reality. For those who have confronted this situation,

empathy for fellow patients comes easily. For those not familiar with chronic suffering, we hope that the personal accounts related in this book will kindle greater compassion, respect, and understanding—particularly for sufferers of Lyme disease.

This book presents the stories of patients who contracted Lyme disease and who were willing to share the lessons they learned with our readers. Their personal stories shed greater light on the common obstacles to proper diagnosis and treatment for this disease. Moreover, these stories are filled with hope and help for those just starting their journey toward healing.

How a person approaches the obstacles to healing depends, in part, on his experiences and outlook on life and, also, a willingness to take charge of his own healthcare. In the case of chronic Lyme disease, which has a unique niche in medical controversy, uncommon burdens are heaped upon the sufferer. In the following pages, fourteen patients relate how they faced the challenges of chronic Lyme disease from their unique perspectives.

When we began searching for interviewees, we found people with Lyme disease from all walks of life and of all ages who wanted their stories to be heard. We were honored by those who wanted to participate and regret that we only had room to showcase a handful of experiences. Those who responded to our call wanted to spread the word about what they had gone through in hopes that it might help others who were new to the illness or felt lost to it. They wanted to let fellow sufferers know they were not alone and that, perhaps, they might learn from the advice offered. Some patients said they wanted a book that would show their loved ones, their friends, and the public in general that their suffering was validated by the common experiences of others.

The individuals interviewed wanted to forewarn readers about the difficulties in obtaining competent medical help. They hoped others could walk in their shoes, for just a little while, to see what it was like to navigate through an indifferent and often abusive medical arena while suffering with frightening symptoms. Over and over again, patients related how the medical profession was unwilling to regard Lyme disease as a chronic disorder that was not always cured with a few weeks of antibiotics. Patients related what they did to survive after they were essentially abandoned by a rigid, medical system that would not flex more than its standard guidelines would allow.

Lyme disease is caused by spiral-shaped bacteria (spirochetes called Borrelia burgdorferi). These organisms are transmitted by small, hard-bodied ticks: the Western black-legged tick (Ixodes pacificus) in the West, and the black-legged tick (Ixodes scapularis) elsewhere, primarily in eastern North America, the Midwest, and states extending to Texas. Other ticks, such as the lone star tick (Amblyomma americanum) and the American dog tick (Dermacentor variabilis) possibly may be linked to transmission.

White-footed mice and deer are the most common hosts for the illness. When humans venture into places where infected hosts and vectors (ticks) live, they increase their chances of becoming inadvertent tick targets. While other insects have been hypothesized to transmit the disease, the primary vector is the hard-bodied tick.

Gestational transmission (mother to fetus) of Lyme disease has been observed. The organism is also able to survive blood processing procedures, and so, the Red Cross will not accept blood from chronic Lyme disease sufferers. Blood donations are only accepted if a patient is treated and remains symptom-free for a year. Other modes of spreading the disease, such as through sexual transmission or breast feeding, need further evidence to substantiate any personal claims and the current, limited research data.

The disease was first formally recognized in

Connecticut in the mid-1970's, and named after Lyme, one of three communities where the disease was observed. Polly Murray, a mother whose family was afflicted with the illness, was instrumental for getting the disease recognized by the medical community. The organism was named after Dr. Willy Burgdorfer, who identified the bacterial cause of the illness in 1981.

Today, Lyme disease and other tick-borne illnesses are among the fastest growing infections in the United States. Cases that were reported to the Centers for Disease Control and Prevention (CDC), from 2000 to 2004, averaged around 20,000 a year. Reported cases underestimate the actual prevalence of illness, and for Lyme disease, the accepted value is around 10 times this figure. About 200,000 cases per year, then, may more closely reflect the actual incidence. Lyme disease has been reported in all states except Montana, but the disease is reported most frequently in the northeast, mid-Atlantic, north central, and west coast states. The disease has been found on all continents.

Following a tick bite, the first sign of Lyme disease may be a rash at the site of the bite. If a doctor recognizes the rash, he can diagnose and treat the illness immediately. This rash, called erythema migrans (EM), however, may go unnoticed or may not appear at all in—arguably—about half of those exposed. It may appear as a bull's-eye rash, but other forms do occur, and not all physicians are aware of the variations. Additional EM's may also appear once the organism disseminates (spreads) throughout the body. The rash can last for a month or longer and go away on its own, but that does not mean the infection is gone. The Lyme spirochetes multiply and move to different locations in the body within days of a bite and even before a rash develops. Next, flu-like symptoms, such as joint pains, fever, and chills usually occur. This stage may go unnoticed as well, or it may be dismissed as merely the flu by both patient and clinician alike.

If recognized and treated early and adequately, the illness most often appears to resolve without complications. When the infection is not stopped early, the bacteria disseminate further throughout the body. More symptoms can arise, such as a stiff neck, severe fatigue, numbness and tingling, severe headaches, heart palpitations, visual problems, migrating joint pains, enlarged lymph glands, and facial palsy. Muscles, joints, tendons, and organs such as the heart, liver, lungs, kidneys, and bladder may be affected, but not in every person. Cognitive problems and psychiatric disorders may also occur

A person with Lyme disease may exhibit many symptoms or only a few. Symptoms can worsen steadily or come and go (relapse and remit). A patient may be told his illness is all in his head when the doctor cannot find a ready explanation. Because the symptoms are common to other disorders, misdiagnoses do occur, and can include multiple sclerosis, rheumatoid arthritis, fibromyalgia, and other illnesses.

Lyme disease is mired in controversy and medical divisions, and the story is long and ongoing. Controversy and contention are not unusual in medicine by any means. In this book, however, we present the human consequences of patients who were caught in the middle of this medical quagmire.

The controversy begins with the question of how to properly diagnose a case of Lyme disease. Prompt diagnosis is essential to minimize any long-term consequences of delayed treatment. Unless a patient presents with the rash typically associated with early Lyme disease—and many do not—he enters the realm of testing.

Many patients encounter their first obstacle to diagnosis when they are tested for Lyme disease. Heavy and unquestioning reliance on testing—often to the complete exclusion of other clinical parameters—can lead to ruling out infection prematurely. The actual bacteria are not commonly evaluated in these assays. Antibodies are usually checked to see if the immune system responded to the infection. If immune function, however, is somehow compromised by a condition or drug, then the results can be a false negative (a result that reads negative when the disease is present).

Inaccuracy, inconsistency from lab to lab, and technical complications compound the problems in testing. A two-step testing procedure is also recommended. Unfortunately, many patients have Lyme totally discounted at the first step in this process. As a result, Western blotting, the second and more exacting test, is usually withheld from the patient even if he requests it. More importantly, test results are only a part of the entire clinical workup. Responding to the widespread misuse of Lyme disease tests, the FDA has cautioned physicians against using tests exclusively to diagnose Lyme disease. The practice, however, remains common.

Patients face additional problems with diagnosis. Since the current, valid Lyme tests are far from perfect, many ill patients looking exclusively for a Lyme diagnosis often turn to unsubstantiated tests to give them a positive result. This increasingly common practice, enabled by many individuals on the Internet, is confusing and dangerous to patients. With a staggering amount of information readily available, an individual searching for answers has a difficult job trying to decide what is worthy of consideration and what is not.

The chasm of professional and medical opinion continues to widen over the most effective treatment medicines and durations of therapy. The overwhelming conventional approach (Infectious Disease Society of America guidelines) is to treat for about a month or so with antibiotics. If the patient is still ill past a predetermined drug cut-off date, ongoing infection is generally dismissed as a likely cause. As a result, additional antibiotic therapy is usually withheld even if progress was made during therapy. High treatment failures of around one-third are repeatedly reported in the literature [1-7] following this conventional, limited antibiotic treatment protocol. Frequently, a patient is labeled with post-Lyme syndrome when he continues to remain ill. This label implies that all infection is gone even though laboratory tests cannot prove this assumption.

Despite 'adequate' antibiotic therapy, persisting infection has been observed in some research studies. However, the majority of physicians view ongoing infection as unlikely in chronic Lyme disease. They believe that further antibiotic treatment is of little or no benefit. While other factors, such as immune dysfunction, may play a role, the unexplained high failure rate of the conventional approach is a major flaw that doctors usually downplay. Other tick-borne diseases may also be found in a Lyme disease patient and complicate the picture. The chronically ill patient can then find himself with a questionable diagnostic label, or he may remain in a diagnostic limbo, unsure of what is actually going on. Frequently, he may be written off as simply having some sort of psychological disorder.

If a patient wishes to be treated with antibiotics in a manner that is determined by his medical response and not by a predetermined cut-off date, he must again fly in the face of convention. The tools he must employ are his wits, common sense, refusal to accept a poorly defined fate, and hope. Usually with no medical background, he must boldly enter the territory of medical authority and learn to fight for his life.

In the following pages are the unvarnished stories of people of diverse backgrounds and occupations, and the details of their struggles with disease, doctors, and a medical system that has been labeled as the best in the world. As patient after patient is forced to grapple with the best way to get help, more questions than answers arise, not only about this particular disease but about the way the medical system is organized to deal with complex medical situations.

Another common thread that runs throughout the stories is of people helping each other. Again and again, patients ultimately obtained competent help through the assistance of others who experienced the disease themselves or who knew someone who had. When the medical hierarchy (medical professionals, insurance companies, and HMO's) failed, the kindness of normal human beings stepped in to guide the way.

As a former support group leader for a decade and a former Lyme disease patient, I can vouch for the necessary element of laymen helping each other in medical matters. The stories presented here, while personal and unique in that respect, are not to be considered rare. With over 10 years of listening to patient and family stories, and after having personally endured both the disease and the medical establishment, I can state that the stories presented are representative of the trials faced by those with this chronic illness.

This book is designed to make the reader think— not only about what the patients had to endure—but also about the quality of medical care they received. The stories should introduce a basic understanding of the disease and its progression, and it should also alert the reader to common obstacles to proper diagnosis and treatment as described by the patients. This book is nonpolitical. No analysis of the politics of Lyme disease or of the medical healthcare system is expressly implied, offered, or endorsed by the authors in *any* part of this book. The authors hold a neutral position with regard to these complex issues and have only related what the patients and their families have presented as accurate histories of their experiences with Lyme disease.

Rita L. Stanley, Ph.D., Portland, Oregon, September 2005

References

1. Asch ES, Bujak DI, Weiss M, Peterson MG, Weinstein A. Lyme disease: an infectious and postinfectious syndrome. *J.Rheumatol* 1994; 21(3): 454-461.

2. Logigian EL, Kaplan RF, Steere AC. Chronic neurologic manifestations of Lyme disease. *N. Engl. J. Med.* 1990; 323 (21): 1438-1444.

3. Pfister HW, Preac-Mursic V, Wilske B, Schielke E, Sorgel F, Einhaupl KM. Randomized comparison of ceftriaxone and cefotaxime in Lyme neuroborreliosis. *J. Infect. Dis.* 1991; 163 (2): 311-318.

4. Shadick NA, Phillips CB, Logigian EL et al. The long-term clinical outcomes of Lyme disease: A population-based retrospective cohort study. *Ann. Intern. Med.* 1994;121(8): 560-567.

5. Shadick NA, Phillips CB, Sangha O et al. Musculoskeletal and neurologic outcomes in patients with previously treated Lyme disease. *Ann. Intern. Med.*1999; 131(12): 919-926.

6. Treib J, Fernandez A, Haass A, Grauer MT, Holzer G, Woessner R. Clinical and serologic follow-up in patients with neuroborreliosis. *Neurology* 1998; 51(5): 1489-1491.

7. Valesova H, Mailer J, Havlik J, Hulinska D, Hercogova J. Long-term results in patients with Lyme arthritis following treatment with ceftriaxone. *Infection.* 1996; 24(1): 98-102.

Authors' Note

Names used in this book are those of actual individuals who wished to have their stories told, and their written permission was obtained to do so. Some individuals, however, wanted to maintain anonymity, so their characters are identified by pseudonyms they have chosen. Where a pseudonym is used in a story, it will appear in italics the first time. Physicians' names remain private unless they are presented as authors of specific publications and/or they appeared in the public media.

The information contained in this book is for educational purposes only. Discuss your healthcare concerns with an appropriate medical professional. The authors disclaim any responsibility (including negligence) from any person acting, or refraining from acting, on information presented in this book.

Rita L Stanley, Ph.D.
Karen P. Yerges

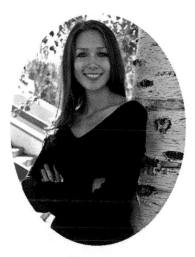

Lauren

From Wisconsin with Love

"If you have knowledge, let others light
their candles at it."

—*Margaret Fuller*

Twelve-year-old Lauren had just finished sixth grade in May 1999, and her summer plans were already arranged. She eagerly looked forward to another fun-filled July vacation in southeastern Wisconsin visiting family and friends she hadn't seen since the previous summer. Reflecting over the many changes that had occurred in her life over recent years, she said, "It was hard to believe that it was only two years ago that I called Wisconsin my home."

The pleasurable memories of her young childhood— rollerblading, swimming, camping, riding bicycles, the theater, county fairs, and countless giggly, sleep-over parties

1

with her girlfriends—endeared her to Wisconsin. Lauren lived an active life seemingly insulated from sorrow. "It was all that I knew until my father became ill with cancer," she recalled.

Lauren's father first became ill when she was seven years old. He was diagnosed with melanoma and underwent numerous procedures, including facial and brain surgery. Lauren was always hopeful that he would get well, but the disease advanced rapidly, and his death seemed inevitable. She witnessed all phases of his decline, including his move to a nursing facility. She stood crying as Hospice care nurses supervised his transfer out of the house and into an ambulance.

Two months later, she stood with her mother alongside his bed on the eve of his death. She stepped closer and clasped his cold hand. Leaning toward his ear she said, "I love you, Daddy." He surrendered his last breath to his Maker, and when Lauren realized this, she broke down in uncontrollable tears. It was her first introduction to the harsh realities of serious illness and premature death.

Lauren's life had been irrevocably altered. Her laughter was never the same after her father's passing. Her times of joy were always shortened because she realized that other girls could go home to their fathers, but she could not. She bore her grief quietly and privately, and only her poetry book knew the secrets of her heart. However, with acceptance and pragmatism, she reasoned that life could only improve from that time forward—after all, there's nothing worse than death, is there?

Blue Mountains of Oregon

About a year later, Lauren's life changed again. Her mother remarried, and her family relocated to the Blue Mountains of northeastern Oregon to start a new life. Of course, she felt mixed emotions leaving Wisconsin and those she loved, but she also realized that life there was devoid of much of the happiness she once enjoyed. She knew her mother was trying to restore some of what they had lost when her father died, so she embraced the hope that her new life would bring them happiness.

They traveled with all their worldly possessions across the Great Plains over a route similar to the Oregon Trail. Defying the snow storms typically forecasted for January, they arrived at their destination after four days of travel. It was well into evening when they pulled to their stop. Lauren was awestruck by the vast, diamond-dotted sky. With her face close to the front windshield and wide open eyes, she saw giant shadows in every direction—mountains—capped with fluorescent looking, blue-white snow. She stepped out of the truck to gaze further at the breathtaking view, and with a sigh, she pondered what her life would be like in this isolated country.

Two days later, she was introduced to her new fifth grade class at the elementary school. She was wary and did not look forward to the smaller school or the chore of building new friendships. As Lauren became acquainted with the rural town, she soon began to realize that she "wasn't in Kansas anymore." The rich amenities and conveniences of her former Wisconsin hometown were starkly absent in this new place, home to only a few residents.

The town's only grocery store was also the post office, the tavern, and the gas station. A spotted mare tied to a hitching post outside was a common sight. The nearest, larger town that offered any amenities now required a special trip referred to as "going to town." At this point, she simply wanted to turn around and go back to Wisconsin. She realized, however, that her past life there was dismantled, and that she had to go forward with acceptance.

Over the next year, Lauren's new friends introduced

her to the pastimes of the great Northwest—riding horses, camping in the mountains, rattlesnake hunting, attending rodeos, and swimming in the rivers. The girl, formerly unaccustomed to solitude, soon discovered the orchestral sounds of crickets and yipping coyotes. She learned to draw some companionship from reading mystery novels, and she returned to writing prose. Slowly, Lauren was transformed. "I have never lived in the country before. I didn't think I'd like it, at first, but it was so beautiful here," she admitted.

Revisiting Wisconsin

Though a fondness for her new Oregon home was forming slowly, summer vacations in Wisconsin were still the highlight of each year. After all, her older sister lived there, as well as her grandparents and other relatives and friends. She looked forward to seeing them all, but by the same token, she always promised her Oregon friends that she would write during her absence. She faithfully wrote and affectionately signed her postcards "from Wisconsin with love."

During one such vacation in July 1999, Lauren experienced the beginning of a medical nightmare that neither she nor her family could ever have anticipated. It all began during a three day visit to her girlfriend's country home in Walworth County. One morning, she woke to find two small, red, itchy spots on her lower left leg. At first she thought they were mosquito bites. However, three days later those two spots grew into well-defined rings, and Lauren felt very ill. She asked her host to take her back to her mother with whom she confided, "Mom, my neck and back hurt so bad—I can hardly move. My eyes are sore, and I'm so tired." Her mother felt her forehead and found that she was very warm despite having taken acetaminophen to bring down her fever.

4

Lauren took a cool bath, but nothing seemed to bring the fever down. Her mother immediately drove her to the emergency room at the local hospital. There Lauren's fever measured 103.3° and was accompanied by chills, fatigue, extreme light sensitivity, headache, nausea, sore muscles, a stiff neck, backaches, and joint pains. Those two, conspicuous bull's-eye marks had grown and looked like erythema migrans (EM) rashes, the classic marker of early Lyme disease.

The attending emergency room (ER) doctor knew that EM rashes were a sure sign of Lyme disease. He felt confident of his suspicions after consulting a large medical book back in his office. Lauren's case looked pretty clear cut but he wanted to get a second opinion from a pediatrician.

As the two physicians examined Lauren's leg, they consulted together over a probable diagnosis. "It appears to be a spider bite," said the pediatrician as he examined the two red rings on Lauren's leg. "What about Lyme disease?" asked the ER physician. "No, I don't think so. Lyme disease is not too common around here. It's probably just an insect bite of some kind," responded the pediatrician. He wrote a prescription for a 21-day course of amoxicillin to cover her localized infection and instructed Lauren to follow up later with her doctor in Oregon.

The emergency room physician, on the other hand, remained unconvinced that Lauren did not have early Lyme disease. He made the following note on his discharge diagnosis: "Fever, etiology to be determined. Rule out Lyme disease."

This was exactly what Lauren's mother intended to do once Lauren could be seen by her family doctor in Oregon. While they were still in Wisconsin, though, Lauren's mother received some advice from her brother-in-law, a pharmacist. He told her that Lyme disease should be treated aggressively with at least six weeks of antibiotics. While amoxicillin was used, her brother-in-law advised her that doxycycline was usually the drug of first choice because it was also effective against several other tick-borne infections. With this information, her mother became concerned about the therapy that Lauren had received. She was eager to follow up on her misgivings with their family practitioner.

Lauren showed minor improvements during the 21 days of treatment. She tried, with difficulty, to resume normal activities for the remainder of her vacation in Wisconsin, but her painful symptoms persisted. "I still had pain in my knees, ankle, and right hand," Lauren noted. "I knew something was really wrong because the medicine didn't seem to be helping me." It was obvious that Lauren's situation needed reevaluation.

As soon as Lauren and her mother returned to Oregon, they went to see their family doctor. Upon examining Lauren, the doctor could still detect the faint bull's-eye marks on her leg, and so he extended the prescription of amoxicillin for five additional weeks. Since the Infectious Disease Society of America (IDSA) guidelines state that early Lyme disease is cured with about a month's worth of doxycycline or amoxicillin, he felt sure Lauren would recover fully. However, that's not how Lauren's story turned out.

Persistent Joint Pains

Throughout the entire treatment time, Lauren continued to complain of intermittent pains in her knees, ankles, and hands. Lauren noted, "My knees became swollen and sore, and moving them for any reason hurt." Oddly, the doctor attributed these symptoms to Osgood-Schlatter disease, a self-limiting condition related to rapid bone growth in adolescents. She was assured that her discomfort was temporary and would stop when she reached her adult height.

It was difficult for Lauren and her mother to believe that her joint pains were not due to Lyme disease, especially in light of the fact that her symptoms seemed to diminish while taking antibiotics. In any event, Lauren was relieved because the antibiotic treatment finally seemed to be working.

This reprieve was short-lived, though. Lauren's therapy ended during the third week of August, shortly before the new school year. Her pains stubbornly persisted and then began to worsen. By the end of September, Lauren's decline in health even showed in her face. Dark purple, or sometimes, red circles began appearing around her eyes. She complained, "I hate how I look, and I don't want anyone to see me like this." She attempted to cover the circles with make-up so that no one would notice at school.

By the end of November, Lauren underwent several blood tests, called Lyme titers or ELISAs (Enzyme-Linked Immunosorbent Assays), indirect tests for the Lyme bacteria (Borrelia burgdorferi). Each time the test came back negative. Lauren and her mother learned later that false negatives on ELISAs were not uncommon. Interpreting Lyme tests was problematic, something even the FDA tried to alert physicians to. Sometimes a patient who receives antibiotic treatment early in the illness has a blunted immune response; antibodies are just not generated in sufficient quantities. As a result, antibody tests can be negative or uncertain. Unaware of these facts, Lauren's physician felt that her condition was under control. However, it was anything *but* under control.

Violent Relapse

On January 4, exactly six months after her initial emergency room visit in Wisconsin, Lauren experienced a new surge of painful symptoms. She awoke that morning with electrifying pains in her right arm and fingers. "It feels like lightning going down my arm and pins in my fingers," she cried.   She also complained of intense pain in her legs, neck, and head.

Her mother began a diary of her symptoms and noted:

January 5, 2000... Complains of pain in fingers, stabbing pain in right arm and shin bones of legs, in neck, and on left side of her head.

January 6, 2000... More of the same pain, stabbing pains in both arms, crying.

Both Lauren and her mother felt helpless and did not understand why she had not been cured by the prescribed therapy.   The following day her pain continued, and she became very weak.   That morning Lauren attempted to shower, but suddenly she called out for help from behind the shower curtain.   Lauren's mother found her huddled and sitting under the spraying water, too weak to stand or to wash herself.   "My arms were so sore that I couldn't lift them to wash my hair.   I became dizzy and thought I was going to fall," Lauren said.   Her mother helped her out of the shower and back into bed.

It seemed fairly obvious at this point that Lauren's treatment had not cured her.   Furthermore, her symptoms were beginning to appear far more complex than she or her mother could imagine.   Lauren's physician was baffled since the therapy was supposed to be curative for Lyme disease, and he began to question whether she had actually been infected.

Lauren's mother became very concerned that their family doctor's doubts might mean the end to her child's treatment.   Her 'mom-sense' told her that Lauren's illness had to be related to those two bull's-eye marks on her leg since that was when all her symptoms began.   Furthermore, she observed that antibiotics appeared to help Lauren somewhat, and when she discontinued taking them, her condition worsened.

For these reasons, Lauren's mother remained firmly focused on Lyme disease as the cause of her daughter's apparent relapse. However, how would she convince their physician? Feeling their doctor's support slipping away, Lauren's mother made an urgent search for someone knowledgeable about Lyme disease—someone who would guide their doctor in the face of this advancing illness.

This situation became an obstacle that even Lauren's mother had not expected. She had to react quickly because her daughter was rapidly worsening. She also had to overcome another obstacle to finding help—the fact that they lived in isolated northeastern Oregon, far from a large city where knowledgeable medical help could more likely be found. All the while, Lauren anxiously kept asking her mother, "What's happening to me?"

Professional Alliance

Faced with so many unanswered questions, Lauren's mother turned to the Internet. During the next two days, she sought basic information on Lyme disease and more importantly, for a support group that could help. After some time-wasting failures, she sent an urgent and pleading email to Rita Stanley, Ph.D., of the Lyme disease support group based at Legacy Good Samaritan Hospital in Portland, Oregon. *It was a shot-in-the-dark,* she thought, but she just had to try.

Dr. Stanley promptly replied and reiterated for clarification what she was told. She suggested some possible explanations for the failure of Lauren's initial treatment. Dr. Stanley said that there were over 100 strains of Lyme spirochetes (cork-screw shaped bacteria) in the U.S. (300 worldwide). Some of these strains responded quickly and fully to treatment while others were more virulent and tougher to eradicate.

She gave some more ideas that Lauren's mom hadn't known. Lyme bacteria may hide in areas of the body (immune-privileged sites) where they cannot be easily attacked by antibiotics or the immune system. If the tick releases a large amount of bacteria while feeding on a victim, not all of them may be killed by the antibiotics prescribed. The bacteria replicate slowly and may even go dormant. They can even change into different forms that can resist antibiotic therapy. These complexities can lead to a situation where the infection is not fully eradicated despite adhering to what should be a curative therapy.

Lauren's mom also learned that ticks sometimes harbor other infections along with the Lyme bacteria (co-infections). Three of the most common are babesiosis, HGE (human granulocytic ehrlichiosis), and HME (human monocytic ehrlichiosis). These diseases can cause severe illness alone. If someone has any of these infections along with Lyme, the Lyme infection can be more difficult to treat. In other words, what looks like one disease may turn out to be several. Whenever that is the case, therapy needs to be geared to a more complete picture of what is going on.

In Lauren's case, one of the first major problems that arose was the Wisconsin pediatrician's lack of knowledge about how prevalent Lyme disease was in his state. He didn't know that the Centers for Disease Control and Prevention (CDC) indicated that his state had high risk areas for the disease. Wisconsin was grouped with 11 other states to account for 95% of all reported cases, and its overall disease incidence was 2.5 times the national average. Fortunately, the ER doctor knew enough to insist that Lauren get reevaluated at home.

At first, the flood of information overwhelmed

Lauren's mother.   She had been led to believe that her daughter had a simple infection that needed a pretty simple solution.   She realized that she had to apply herself to gathering knowledge and to get that information to Lauren's doctor. She decided to ask her physician if Dr. Stanley could help supply information to assist in Lauren's case. When the doctor readily agreed, any anticipated resistance immediately turned to relief.

Hope shed its light upon Lauren at last. Now her mother could more confidently answer Lauren's repeated question, "Will I be all right, Mom?" Feeling quite helpless, Lauren looked to her mother for encouragement every day. Lauren said, "I looked to my mother for comfort and hope. I needed her to tell me I was going to be okay." Her mother reassured her that two very skilled professionals were going to take care of her and that she was going to get well soon.

The Details of Testing

The doctor decided that he would test Lauren's blood again, but in a manner somewhat different than before. This time Dr. Stanley suggested doing ELISAs simultaneously with Western blot assays and to make sure both IgG and IgM antibodies were evaluated. At first, this all sounded very complicated for Lauren's mother to comprehend. She was assured, however, that she was quite capable of understanding the jargon after a bit of an explanation.

The ELISA and Western blot tests are called indirect tests or assays. A direct test would test for the actual organism or parts of it. An indirect one looks for signs of a particular agent that can be readily measured. The particular tests that would be used in Lauren's case check for antibodies.

Simply, antibodies are very specific proteins produced by part of the immune system in response to the presence of specific substances called antigens. In the case of Lyme disease, the bacteria, Borrelia burgdorferi, are the antigens. IgM antibodies are a type that can be found early in infections but, in some cases, may also exist in Lyme disease of long-standing duration. IgG antibodies show up later in the disease process. Both types of antibodies can be measured in both ELISA and Western blot tests.

The ELISA measures a class of antibodies, but the Western blot is much more specific. It reveals antibodies that the body makes to specific areas of the Lyme organism. The results reveal both the number and the type of those antibodies and are reported as bands. The numbers of the bands actually indicate very small units of mass (kilodaltons).

Lauren only had the ELISA run before. This time, she would have the Western blot run at the same time. Admittedly, this approach is not accepted by most practitioners. It differs from the two-tiered, conventional method of doing the Western blot only if the ELISA proves positive. Since Lauren faced a potentially disabling illness, the doctor felt that simply running an additional test would give him a clearer picture of what might be going on.

The testing situation got even more complicated. Knowing the numbers and types of bands in the Western blot test are important so that the disease is not ruled out prematurely. Most labs, however, only report a positive Western blot based on very stringent criteria. In order for a positive result, five significant bands are needed for the IgG test and three for the IgM. The doctor knew that the presence of any significant banding was an essential clue about infection, so he would ask the lab to give him the exact banding results.

The physician also learned that above all, the test results should not be used alone to rule in or rule out a diagnosis of Lyme disease. The FDA issued a warning to tell doctors, "The tests should be used only to support a clinical diagnosis of Lyme disease and should **never** be the primary basis for making diagnostic or treatment decisions. Diagnosis should be based on a patient history, which includes symptoms and exposure to the tick vector and physical findings" (FDA Medical Bulletin; summer, 1999).

In addition to more fully evaluating Lauren for Lyme disease, she was also going to be tested for a few co-infections. Tests would be run for the two most common types of ehrlichiosis: human monocytic ehrlichiosis (HME) and human granulocytic ehrlichiosis (HGE).

Ehrlichiosis is caused by rickettsia-like bacteria (organisms related to Rocky Mountain spotted fever) that invade white blood cells. The most common symptoms are sudden, high fever, tiredness, major muscle aches, severe headache, and in some cases, a rash which appears 3 to 16 days after a tick bite. This disease can make it harder to fight off other infections as well. Since Lauren experienced a spiking fever very early in her illness, it seemed logical to order a test for the disease.

Blood Tests

Lauren's physician ordered the tests for the tick-borne infections through the Oregon Department of Public Health. Meanwhile, the arthritic pain in Lauren's lower body became a daily experience. She limped and every movement was slow and deliberate like that of a geriatric patient. She explained, "I felt like an old woman, and I couldn't run or jump anymore. My friends at school expected me to hang out with them, but I got too tired and stayed behind in the lunchroom. That's when I began to use my lunch hours as study periods."

Finally, on January 24, 2000, her doctor received the blood test results. The report read negative for Lyme disease and for ehrlichiosis. How could this be? *Something must be wrong*, Lauren's mother thought. In fact, something was wrong—it turned out that the doctor's orders for Western blotting had been ignored by the Health Department. Only Lyme ELISAs had been done; it was another waste of precious time.

Dr. Stanley quickly advised Lauren's mother to reorder the same tests and submit the samples to another lab where all bands for the Lyme Western blot would be reported, and to make sure that the handling of the test samples was exacting. Simple mishandling of samples or allowing the samples to sit for too long without temperature control could result in false negative results. This time, the tests would be done as ordered and with an eye out for anything that might interfere with getting accurate answers.

With both Lauren's mother and the doctor closely monitoring every step in the process, Lauren's blood was drawn on a Monday and shipped express to the lab so that testing could be completed before the week's end. On the following Monday, February 7, the results of those tests came back—Western blot positive for Lyme disease and positive for one type of ehrlichiosis. It was bittersweet news, but finally Lauren had laboratory confirmation of what she was battling.

School Challenges

Eight months had passed since the tick bite, and the disease had disseminated throughout Lauren's body. She now had disabling arthritic symptoms in many of her joints. Her once spindly knees were swollen and round, and they ached terribly with every movement. It took all the courage she had to attend 7th grade at public school.

Early each morning, she caught the bus in front of her country home and rode it to school. For most kids, those first three steps entering the bus took nothing more than a hop, skip, or jump. For Lauren, it was like climbing a mountain,

14

each step taken slowly and deliberately. She used the hand rail to help her up, and then she plopped down on the nearest seat. Climbing the stairs at school was particularly difficult for her, so at times, friends would carry her books up and down the stairs. At five foot three inches tall and 110 pounds, Lauren found it hard to even lift her own body weight. With the added weight of heavy textbooks, what used to be an easy exercise turned into an overwhelming burden.

Before long, she routinely came home with an empty backpack. At first, her mother questioned her, thinking she might be neglecting her studies. After all, she used to carry at least 20 pounds on her back. Lauren explained, "My school books were too heavy for me to carry around. It hurt my knees to climb the school stairs or the bus steps with that kind of weight."

Her lower body, particularly her knees, was in constant pain, and any weight bearing exercise increased her misery. Soon it became impossible for her to participate in any running exercises, a requirement in her physical education class. Lauren's doctor wrote a note that excused her from all activities involving her lower body. Despite this, she did not look forward to presenting the note to her teacher.

Her teacher read the doctor's excuse and then looked at her as if searching to see some sign of this disease she was supposed to have. Clearly irritated by the note, the teacher firmly reminded her that she *would perform* all the other nonexempt activities. "I was so embarrassed because some of the other kids heard this and started to tease me, saying I was just being lazy and faking it," she recalled. Lauren came home many days discouraged and in despair. Her physical suffering was burden enough without the added emotional stress caused by such a lack of compassion.

Lauren was determined to make it through 7th grade despite feeling like she had been "run over by a truck."

Pushing through her pain, she summoned her internal resolve and finished her homework during study hall and lunch hour simply to avoid lugging a heavy load home. "I didn't want to miss school or get lower grades because of being sick. I wasn't going to let this disease beat me," she said. To succeed in her goals, she needed to keep to a disciplined schedule at school and at home.

Each day when she returned home from school, she ate an early dinner, took a warm bath to relieve her pain, and resigned herself to bed. There she slept from 4:30 pm until morning. This was so unlike the Lauren her family used to know, a girl who never went to bed before ten o'clock. Now her activities were confined strictly to school and to necessary sleep.

Treatment and Herxheimer-like Reactions

The doctor devised a plan for Lauren to treat both Lyme disease and the ehrlichiosis. Rather than treating her for about a month with antibiotics, which is recommended by the Infectious Disease Society of America (IDSA), he decided on an open-ended course of therapy. The selection of medicine and the duration of treatment would be based on Lauren's response. Her therapy would be modified when necessary and stopped when her symptoms had abated.

Lauren started to take the antibiotic, doxycycline, which treats both diseases. The medicine presented some challenges of its own; Lauren experienced nausea and some diarrhea. Determined not to let this thwart her treatment plan, she and her mother experimented with different foods and eating times. Eventually, they found a routine that minimized the nausea. "I still felt sick every morning, but the feeling usually went away by lunch hour. I was so glad I didn't have to run laps or play any sports in P.E. That made it a lot easier for me to make it through the day," she said.

Lauren also took generous doses of acidophilus, a friendly bacteria, to help maintain her gastrointestinal health.

Finding ways to alleviate the discomforts associated with occasional flare-ups was a learn-as-you-go experience. "I seemed to feel a little better if I stayed warm, so I took warm baths when my joints hurt real bad. I also dressed in warm pajamas and socks and went to bed to sleep and stay warm. Ibuprofen seemed to help with joint pain, too," Lauren explained.

After six weeks, Lauren started on another antibiotic, Biaxin. During this time, the physician carefully monitored her progress to see what modifications were necessary. He understood that not all patients responded the same to a particular medication. While these two antibiotics were hoped to benefit Lauren, he didn't have any preconceived ideas and was willing to work with what would most benefit his patient. He made sure that liver tests were performed regularly to assure that Lauren's liver stayed healthy throughout the ordeal.

Lauren was forewarned that she might experience a temporary worsening of symptoms when she first started taking antibiotics or when she was changed to another type. The name given to this response was the Jarisch Herxheimer-like reaction or, in shortened form, a Herxheimer-like reaction. Getting worse before getting better was a hard concept for her to understand.

The doctor explained that when a large number of Lyme spirochetes were killed off all at once—at the beginning of treatment or when a new antibiotic was introduced—the immune system produced a lot of inflammatory products. These substances could make her symptoms worse for a time. As treatment advanced, fewer bacteria would be killed, and so the production of these harsh substances would diminish. She would then start to feel better.

Lauren wanted to know why this experience had

such an odd name. Originally, the name came from two doctors—Jarisch and Herxheimer—who described what they saw in patients who had syphilis. When these patients were treated with penicillin, they got worse at the beginning of treatment. This was caused by a large, sudden release of toxins from the killed bacteria. When the toxins were eliminated from their bodies, the patients got better. The doctors named the phenomenon after themselves, the Jarisch-Herxheimer reaction. Since the cause of the reaction is somewhat different in Lyme disease, "-like" is added to the end of the doctors' names.

Neurological Involvement

Lauren found that her illness had advanced and affected her central nervous system. One morning, Lauren's mother gave her customary wake-up call through Lauren's bedroom door. Ten minutes later, no noise came to indicate that she was up and about. Then from the bedroom, her faint voice cried out, "Mom! Help! I can't move." When Lauren's mother found her, she was lying still on her back in bed. Lauren explained, "Mom, I can't move my legs!" She had feeling in her legs, but she could not move them. Lauren was very frightened.

The paralysis persisted for about five minutes, and then she could move her legs and sit up in bed with her mother's help. She looked at her mother and asked, "What was that? What just happened?" Her mother didn't know what to tell her, but she reassured Lauren that she would find out. Not long after this bizarre event, Lauren and her mother viewed a Lyme video borrowed from the Good Samaritan Hospital's video library. The video explained that Lyme patients with neurological involvement may experience what is called Lyme induced post-sleep paralysis. This temporary paralysis of the limbs occurs just as the patient wakes from normal sleep. Lauren and her mother instantly recognized this symptom as the one Lauren experienced earlier.

Lauren also developed other neurological problems that included palsy and seizures. Her mother's entries in her medical diary described the symptoms:

May 16, 2000...Right hand shaking uncontrollably. Needle-poking pain in both heels and in ribs. Comes on suddenly without notice. Lasts 5-20 seconds per episode. Hard to lift arms. Pain on underside of the arm. Pain in finger joints. Heavy eyelids.

There was no doubt that Lauren's nervous system was under aggressive attack.

Recovery

Lauren continued taking her antibiotics, and she slowly began to improve as the months passed. Her symptoms got better progressively until they ceased altogether in July 2000. The numbness in her limbs went away, and the paralysis and shaking incidences ceased. Her energy level rose, and she began to forsake her bedroom for the living room. She began sleeping less and gradually gained back her mental and physical abilities. Pain was no longer a constant companion. "There were days when I thought I'd never feel this well again. I'm so grateful for the help I received from my doctor and Dr. Stanley," Lauren said.

When she reached a symptom-free state, her doctor wanted to reassure Lauren's family that if she relapsed, antibiotic therapy would immediately resume. Lauren felt some security in the thought that her future health status would take into account her Lyme disease history. She knew that no test could show that all the bacteria were gone from her system, so her symptoms would be the guide to any problems that might arise in the future.

On September 11, 2000, Lauren finished her antibiotic treatment. As much as she wanted to celebrate this occasion, she felt a guarded sense of optimism. Having relapsed nine months earlier, she knew it was premature to say that she was out of the woods. Only time would tell if her treatment had been sufficient to keep her well.

A Change of Lauren's Choosing

Good health followed Lauren into the 2000-2001 school year. Except for a bout of mild swelling in her knees, she was pain-free and active again. Her appearance was healthy—her large, white smile was free of the previous year's orthodontics, and she was two inches taller. She felt like a new person in many ways, and she was happy again.

Lauren's life, up until then, had undergone changes over which she had no control. Her father's death, her mother's remarriage, their relocation to Oregon, and her struggles with Lyme disease were life-changing events. She adapted and survived, but now she wanted to have a voice in her own future. Her last school year had been very challenging because she had to defend herself from verbal abuse and ignorance on top of coping with her illness.

What if she relapsed during 8th grade? Lauren did not want to face another year in public school sick with Lyme disease. She chose to leave the public school system and enrolled with a local home school agency. Lauren felt confident that she would excel in this self-motivated program, and so, for the first time, she made a change of her own choosing.

It turned out to be a good choice for Lauren. During the ensuing high school years, she remained healthy with no relapses. Her home schooling situation allowed her to immerse herself into many ambitious experiences that offered unique interactions with her community. She said, "I studied journalism for three years. The personal interviewing process provided me with a wider scope of social contact and learning experiences. I wrote human interest stories, medical and career choice stories, and articles highlighting small businesses and the arts. I was very busy in this class."

Lauren's articles were regularly published in a local newspaper with a circulation of about 5,000 copies weekly. The editor later honored her contribution to his paper and presented her with an award plaque that read, "Home School Writer of the Year—2001." She also received scholarships for her journalism from community professionals.

By the time Lauren finished her junior year of home schooling, she was an honor roll student with a 3.82 grade point average and 23 transcripted high school credits. She was ahead of her game and even took a few university courses before she graduated in March of 2005.

Around classes, she worked two part-time jobs including a job waitressing. She had the stamina and health to perform well at all her activities. At the end of the day, her only special requests included a good foot rub and a soft bed.

With restored health, Lauren also took up snowboarding with her friends. "I've biffed hard a few times, but I really enjoy this winter sport," she said. For Lauren, the world has become her oyster, and she has the health and strength to enjoy it.

Back on the Horse

No grass grows under Lauren's feet these days. She doesn't like to dwell on, or even look back at, her time with Lyme disease. Though she is forward thinking, she will occasionally glance over her shoulder just to see how far she has come. It is an exercise in appreciation and a review of the lessons that suffering taught her.

She won the battle for her life despite the eight month delay in correct diagnosis and treatment. She experienced the obstacles of misdiagnosis, false negative test results, and an overlooked co-infection, all-too-common failures in the medical management of Lyme disease. Her doctor chose to think beyond the most widely accepted diagnostic and treatment guidelines. He ran a few more tests to clarify Lauren's diagnosis, and he wouldn't accept a predetermined time for stopping medication when his patient was clearly still ill.

Despite her delay in treatment and inadequate early treatment, Lauren was still able to achieve a symptom-free state of health. Her success had much to do with the fact that she received help within a time frame that allowed for full recovery. She also had a strong parental advocate who found knowledgeable medical professionals to carry out the management of her treatment.

From Lauren's perspective, her experience with Lyme disease gave her added appreciation for those who suffer from serious, debilitating diseases. She remembered what it appeared to be like for her father during his excruciating illness, but that knowledge came to her only as a close observer. In her early teens, she learned what severe, chronic suffering personally *felt* like. She learned the meaning of and need for compassion, and it transformed her into a mature and caring young woman.

Today Lauren has moved on with her life, as one would expect, but not without the life-changing imprint that Lyme disease left on her. One thing hasn't changed—she still travels to Wisconsin to see family and friends. "It symbolizes the best and the worst in my life. It holds memories of a very happy childhood, but also, of the unbearable sorrows of my father's death and the source of my Lyme disease," she confided.

Nonetheless, her Northwestern upbringing taught her to "get back on the horse," and she did. She is a survivor, and she doesn't fear going back to the place where these tragedies occurred. It is part of her history and who she is today. Through it all, one thing has not changed. Whenever she visits Wisconsin, she doesn't hesitate to send her Oregon friends post cards—affectionately signed, as always—"from Wisconsin with love."

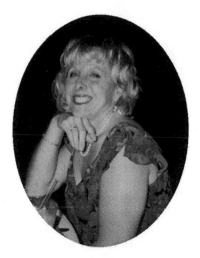

Linda

On the Front Line

"In all things it is better to hope than to despair."
—*Johann Wolfgang von Goethe*

In this uncertain world, there are many threats to health and life. Unbeknownst to Linda Rinaldi, 38, of Terryville, Connecticut, a very real danger hid nearby in a grassy field just across the road from her country home.

On a breezy spring day in 1990, Linda and her two young children, Jamie, 10, and Bethany, 7, went to fly kites in that grassy field, never thinking for a moment that peril was lying in wait there. Admittedly, Linda had never given much thought to ticks or to Lyme disease, despite the fact that Lyme disease had been found in Connecticut in the mid 1970s and subsequently named after a Connecticut town where an early disease cluster appeared. "Lyme disease was something that you vaguely heard of but never thought anything about, especially back then," Linda explained.

Far from thinking of such dangers, Linda immersed herself in her busy family life. She was a dedicated wife and working mother, who balanced her family affairs with her job as a medical transcriptionist at the local hospital. "I always considered myself [to be] a pretty happy and stable person. I had a good life, great husband, and two wonderful children. I was very involved in all their activities, school, sports, and dance [lessons]; and I enjoyed every minute of it," Linda said.

Linda had never had any notable medical problems and was the picture of health until May of 1990, when she experienced a sudden onset of flu-like symptoms. "I was supposed to take my children on a bus trip to the Statue of Liberty with friends of ours. The day before, [however], I became very ill with what I thought was the flu, but worse than any flu I had [ever] experienced."

This extraordinary "flu" lasted three weeks, quickly exhausting all of Linda's employee sick-time benefits. The rest of the time spent recuperating was without pay. She was anxious to get well and become a wage earner again, but then she began to notice an alarming change in her vision. "Everything I looked at was vibrating, almost as if [I was] looking through heat rising on a hot summer day. I also had severe light sensitivity," she explained.

Search for a Diagnosis

Linda had consulted with her primary care doctor twice during the first week of her illness because she sensed there was something seriously wrong with her. She had never experienced any flu like this before. It wasn't the low grade fever or the 10 pound weight loss that alarmed her. No, those things could happen with the flu, and Linda knew that. However, she also realized that her difficulty standing up and her impaired spatial perceptions were definitely not typical flu symptoms. In addition to those strange symptoms, she noticed that she could not move one hand very well.

She recalled the moment the latter symptom became very obvious. "A friend came over to get a check from me for the Parent Teacher Association. It took me about five minutes to write out the check. I couldn't make my hand do what I wanted it to do."

Consequently, on Linda's first consultation with her doctor, she told him there was something wrong with her and that it wasn't the flu. The doctor, however, thought that one week was too soon to conclude that this illness was anything else, so he adopted a wait and see approach and encouraged Linda to come back if she did not feel better in another week.

During the second week of illness at home, Linda happened to watch a television program about Lyme disease on the *Sally Jesse Raphael Show*. The information presented on this show was novel because very few programs, at that time, highlighted the topic of the disorder. As Linda listened intently to the testimony of the patient guests, she heard about symptoms that were strangely similar to her own. Could it be possible that she had this infection? After all, Connecticut surely was on the front line as far as investigating early clusters of the disease in children. Certainly, physicians would be knowledgeable about all of this, wouldn't they? It had been a long time since the first publication naming the disease after Lyme, Connecticut, in 1977, so surely much more would be known by now—or so Linda thought.

Three weeks into her illness, she once again saw her primary care doctor. She asked him if he thought she could possibly have Lyme disease. She felt certain that this physician was qualified to answer her question because he was an infectious disease specialist. He responded by asking Linda if her knees hurt, and she said no. Based upon this fact, he concluded that if she wasn't feeling pain in her knees, then she did not have Lyme disease. He did say, however, that if the flu-like illness did not go away, then she might have chronic fatigue syndrome. Linda requested some information on that disorder, but the doctor did not have any literature on hand at the time.

Frustrated over not being taken seriously, Linda decided to take the initiative and address her persisting visual disturbances with an ophthalmologist. After examining her eyes, this doctor asked the nurse to summon Linda's husband into the office for a serious discussion. The doctor informed Linda and her husband that he detected a condition known as papilledema, swelling of the optic nerve. This condition was most commonly caused by increased intracranial pressure and was very frequently accompanied by headache. The doctor was puzzled that Linda did not have a headache. Nonetheless, he urgently advised Linda to go to the hospital for an emergency spinal tap procedure and a CAT scan of her head to determine the cause of this pressure.

Linda's CAT scan proved unremarkable, but the spinal tap did reveal some abnormalities, leading the physician to a diagnosis of resolving viral meningitis. "[It was] resolving because I had been sick already for three weeks," Linda explained. Then about a week later, all of her symptoms abated. Linda, while puzzled at this turn of events, was deeply grateful to have seemingly regained her health.

Reoccurrence

Linda returned to her job in June 1990, happy and relieved to be feeling pretty much like herself again. It had been a harrowing four weeks, but it was time to move on, she thought. "Everything was great until September of 1990 when the visual symptoms came back," Linda said. She had another spinal tap performed, but this time, no abnormalities were noted. Puzzled, she requested a Lyme disease test, but those results proved negative as well.

Shortly after the vision problems reappeared, Linda also noticed other symptoms which she felt were bizarre. She experienced rib pain, shooting pains in her legs, and a strange feeling that her arms were not attached to her body. In addition to these new symptoms, she had what she described as a constant and severe pressure in the back of her head. "Sometimes it was so bad that I felt my head shaking, my teeth chattering, and I could not make a fist without having jerky movements of my hands. The feeling [head pressure] was somewhat like having a brick tied to the top of your head," Linda said.

From September 1990 until March 1991, Linda saw five different physicians. "Some really tried to figure it all out, and several were downright hostile." All of these consultations were frustrating to Linda because no one was able to diagnose her illness. It was, after all, strangely complex; and in defaulting to helplessness, some physicians dismissed her complaints by suggesting her illness had a mental origin. For Linda, such conjecture was both cruel and terribly demoralizing. Linda summed it up this way, "When a doctor doesn't know what is wrong with you, [he may try] to make it look like it is 'all in your head.'"

One of the five physicians she consulted suggested that she might be "feeling sympathy pains" for her father, who had just had cardiac bypass surgery. Noticing Linda's disapproving facial response, the doctor dismissed that theory and then asked her if she was having any marital trouble. This line of questioning was way off target and a costly waste of time for Linda. All she wanted was to become well again.

Neurological Involvement

From January through March of 1991, Linda took a leave of absence from work to address her ongoing illness. The head pressure that she had felt since September 1990 was worsening. She was also experiencing disorientation and surrealism of her surroundings. "I couldn't find my way anywhere, and I constantly felt like I was living inside a clear plastic bag."

Then neurological problems appeared on the right side of her face and in her right arm. She experienced constant numbness and tingling in these areas. When her right eyelid began to droop, she became frightened and decided immediately to see a neurologist.

She selected a neurologist from a large state teaching hospital in Connecticut. While being examined by him, she related how her illness had begun with flu-like symptoms and then had expanded to include new and disturbing symptoms over a few months' time. Intrigued by the complexity and diversity of her problem, the doctor listened intently. However, because her medical history sounded so unusual, he dismissed it as a psychiatric disorder instead of a physical disease. The neurologist told her that if she did not get over this obsession with her "flu-like symptoms," she should seek psychiatric counseling.

Frustrated over his lack of knowledge and scared that she still had no one to help her, Linda collected herself and responded, "There is something *physically* wrong with me, and I will go see every doctor in Connecticut if I have to." With that said, she began her search for knowledgeable medical help.

A Friend's Recommendation

In March, one of Linda's friends told her about a

competent doctor who practiced in a nearby town. Having nothing to lose, Linda made an appointment with him for a clinical evaluation. The physician listened to her medical history, performed a physical exam, and then ordered blood tests for Lyme disease. The results of the tests came back and confirmed a diagnosis of Lyme disease. Of all the physicians in Connecticut with whom Linda could have consulted, she was finally referred to someone who had a good working knowledge of Lyme disease. "It was a miracle that literally saved my life. I could have gone to just about every doctor in the state and not one would have known what was wrong with me," Linda said.

Feeling as though she had just been vindicated, Linda took her diagnosis and test results to the human resource department at her place of employment. Finally, she had something to justify her leave of absence for the past three months. It wasn't a psychiatric disorder that talk therapy could relieve, as erroneously suggested by the neurologist from the state teaching hospital. Rather, Linda suffered from a very real, disseminated bacterial infection affecting her nervous system that could include progressive neuropsychiatric involvement.

Treatment was started during the last week in March with an antibiotic called Suprax, a cephalosporin. Linda explained, "After taking Suprax, my symptoms got better but were not gone. I was able to return to work in the beginning of April." However, after two months, she became very ill again. "We were on a three day weekend and had to come home. I couldn't even sit up," said Linda. Fearing that perhaps this bad reaction was evidence that Suprax would not be curative for her and that she might worsen further, she decided to stop her treatment altogether. "I did fairly well over the summer. I still had head pressure, but then in September 1991, I started getting symptoms [again]," Linda recalled.

Relapse

By October, all of Linda's previous alarming symptoms reappeared along with the introduction of some new ones. Again, she took a leave of absence from work for a few months. She said, "I was now having severe symptoms of disorientation, living in a fog, head pressure, and very severe anxiety to the point where I would pace the floors. I had extreme sound sensitivity and couldn't even be in the same room when my husband was emptying the dishwasher." Agitated intensely by normal household noises, Linda became even more anxious over her feeling of increasing helplessness. "I was living in mental [torment]."

Additionally, her perception of space and movement was altered by this new attack of symptoms. "I could not even go to the grocery store because I felt like the isles were tipping, the floors were moving, and the fluorescent lights just made everything seem more unreal." This distortion of spatial orientation greatly limited her mobility. She knew she was not going crazy, but it was frightening nonetheless. "The world is a very scary place when you have a brain infection," Linda remarked.

She began to worry that going off antibiotics without consulting her doctor had been a mistake. Alarmed at the severity of her latest neurological symptoms, she returned to her doctor. He prescribed intravenous (IV) Rocephin, but shortly thereafter, terminated this treatment when Linda developed an allergic reaction to it.

Then Linda's doctor prescribed a second IV antibiotic, Claforan. She was admitted into the hospital in November just in case she developed a serious allergic reaction. "At the time, I was having terrible heart palpitations and shortness of breath and had a Holter [heart] monitor placed while I was there. The Claforan IV antibiotic took care of [the heart palpitations]."

Despite some improvement in her condition, she developed an early reaction to the medicine which included fever and rash. The doctor felt her response might have been a Herxheimer-like reaction, so he reduced her dose by half, monitored her condition very closely, and kept her on this drug for six months. She was able to tolerate the treatment well, but many of her symptoms persisted.

Completely discouraged, Linda fell into a severe depression accompanied by suicidal thoughts. "I just wanted to get out of the very sick body and mind I was living in. But I had two children and a husband I desperately loved and did not want to leave them."   Linda admittedly experienced her lowest point during this difficult time, but she had also learned something about mental illness. "This experience made me a truly compassionate person toward anyone who deals with mental illness on a daily basis."

Passage of Time

Linda tried to go back to work despite her physical and mental suffering. "It was really difficult to relate to anything at my job. I was so disoriented, and [I was] experiencing some bizarre symptoms. One day in December, I just walked out the door at work, giving no notice. I just walked out and said, 'I just can't do this anymore.' I was so sick."

Linda went back on Suprax in the spring of 1992, but only for a short time because in April, a new antibiotic, Zithromax, came onto the market. She decided to try it, but she became extremely ill, suffering numerous physical symptoms and mental confusion. Her mental impairment became shockingly obvious to her one day when she became lost trying to drive to her daughter's school to pick her up. She pulled her car over to the side of the street and cried. "I didn't know how to get there," Linda explained.

Linda's Herxheimer-like reaction persisted for a couple of days. Then to her great surprise, most of her symptoms lifted for the first time since she became ill in 1990. "I felt like I was myself again. The fog lifted, all the psychiatric and physical ailments left, and I was on top of the world." For the next four years, Linda enjoyed longer periods of good health with only occasional episodes of severe flare-ups. During this time, her open-ended antibiotic therapy was adjusted according to her needs.

After four years of treatment, when she felt like a "semi-functioning" person, Linda decided that she wanted to help others who were looking for knowledgeable direction in their own fight against Lyme disease. She said, "I kept my focus on getting my name and number out there." After all, it was initially the recommendation of a friend that led her to a doctor who was willing to treat this disease when relatively little was known about it.

Gastrointestinal Affliction

Though Linda felt much better, she did experience occasional vaginal yeast infections, but she treated those successfully with miconazole (Monistat). To control gastrointestinal yeast overgrowth (such as candida), she took daily doses of an acidophilus preparation. As suggested by her physician, she also took daily multi- and B-complex vitamins to support her immune system and other body systems.

Over the years, she had never complained of any gastrointestinal problems often associated with long-term antibiotic use. However, in 1998, a few weeks after she stopped taking Suprax, she was admitted to the hospital for three days of intractable vomiting. Linda explained, "I burped and spit up vile fluids about every 30 seconds, starting about an hour after eating. If I ate a regular meal, I would vomit for a few days. I had to go to the emergency room a few times for this."

Linda underwent a gastric emptying scan, which involved eating radioactive scrambled eggs and then submitting to x-rays every ten minutes to monitor the progress of digestion in her stomach. From the results, Linda was diagnosed with gastroparesis, a condition where the stomach does not contract to digest food and responds to a full stomach by vomiting. Linda was told that the nerve from her brain that signaled her stomach to contract had somehow become dysfunctional.

Considering all the neurological symptoms Linda suffered while chronically ill with Lyme disease, this was another to add to the list. "I could hardly eat anything without a lot of discomfort, but when I started taking Suprax again, those [gastroparesis] symptoms went away," Linda said.

Linda lost a total of 25 pounds from this affliction, weight that she never regained. For Linda, the weight loss was one of the few positives that resulted from this ailment. She felt younger and more energetic. "I do not have the desire to eat very much. I don't have the same cravings for the foods that I used to [eat]. I stay at about the same weight all the time now, weighing one or two pounds less from one year to the next," said Linda.

Only specific antibiotics were effective for Linda's gastroparesis. She noted, "Years ago, before Reglan came out, gastroenterologists treated this condition with antibiotics, but [they] did not know how the [antibiotics] worked, and sometimes they didn't. The macrolides (Zithromax, Biaxin) do nothing for my stomach problem. The cephalosporins do. Suprax was taken off the market for lack of interest, and [so] the doctor and I tried Ceftin. That worked too." From that point on, Linda started taking one dose of Ceftin late each morning to control her stomach discomfort.

Thorough Evaluation

Linda was very concerned that her neurological symptoms might have resulted from damage due to the bacterial infection in her brain, so she asked her doctor if he would agree to order a SPECT brain scan. He agreed since he was equally concerned and especially because she had been diagnosed with gastroparesis. A SPECT or Single Photon Emission Computed Tomography scan allows for visualizing certain functional information about an organ. Both Linda and her doctor were curious to see what it might reveal about her brain.

Linda purposely went off all her antibiotics for five days before the test so that the scan would show her brain in its unmedicated state. All of her former, horrid symptoms returned with a rage when she went off the antibiotics, but she was willing to endure this if it would provide the truest image of her brain's condition. The results of Linda's SPECT brain scan were serious. "It showed hypoperfusion of almost every part of my brain," Linda recalled.

The doctor who viewed and read the SPECT brain scan made the following medical report: "There is considerable hypoperfusion involving frontal, temporoparietal and the majority of the occipital lobes. The far most posterior occipital cortex around the calcarine is preserved. There is also hypoperfusion of the basal ganglia. Cerebellar perfusion is intact. The subcortical white matter also appears to be hypoperfused."

Hypoperfusion is a condition where there is a decrease in the blood flow. When this happens in the brain—and depending on the areas affected—specific systems of the body, as well as, mental, cognitive, and emotional functioning can be adversely impacted. To Linda, that scan was additional proof that her brain had been impaired by Lyme disease.

Since then, Linda has armed herself with that brain

scan and has taken it with her on all her consultations with new physicians. She has made it her practice to describe her Lyme disease history to all new doctors. If any of these doctors exhibit disbelief or apathy, she slips the brain scan out from its protective envelope and provides her proof. For Linda, the days of enduring disbelief, apathy and arrogance are past. Now the responses are uniformly, "Lyme disease can do this to you?"

Coping with Lyme

Linda's personal struggle with Lyme disease has been waged since 1990. The costs in terms of emotional and mental suffering have been substantial. The toll mounts ever further when the economic costs, including hospital bills, doctor bills, and prescription drugs are counted. When times were their toughest, Linda was on Social Security Disability and resorted to buying groceries with her credit card.

The Rinaldi's spent $80,000 of their own money over the years even though insurance picked up 75-80% of the bills. Grateful for the economic aid she did have, Linda said, "I have been luckier than many people in that I haven't had to fight with my insurance [company] to pay for a diagnosis of Lyme disease. I was very fortunate that I was still able to work some at home."

The hospital, where she had been employed in 1990, cooperatively allowed her to work at home as a medical transcriptionist. This was a true blessing because for many years, Linda was unable to work outside the home or even look for a job. Eventually, though, the hospital stopped outsourcing their medical dictations to home workers, and she had to seek other employment.

In 2003, Linda accepted a position as a medical transcriptionist in a doctor's office. While she has been able to handle the responsibilities of this job, it hasn't been easy. "I have a lot of cognitive problems, and I know the people I work with really can't understand. I feel very stupid sometimes. I am always a few seconds slower trying to figure things out. When things go wrong, I have a heck of a time figuring them out again." Obviously, Linda still has challenges that underscore her continuing need for antibiotics.

"As difficult as this is to comprehend—if I go off antibiotics, within three days, I start getting a lot of pressure in the back of my head. [It's] very uncomfortable to the point where I feel like my teeth are chattering, [and my body is] trembling. [There is] numbness on the right side of my face [accompanied by] fogginess and a feeling as if everything around me is surreal. These symptoms come back even after all these years." For the past six years, Linda has been taking Biaxin instead of Zithromax and has seen improvements, but she still lives each day with varying intensities of head pressure located in the back and crown of her head. "Most days are livable," she said.

Still, she is very aware of the constant threat of a relapse as if it hovers over her like a darkened storm cloud. "It is sometimes hard to live with this hanging over my head, wondering what my future will bring if for some reason, I could not take antibiotics," Linda said with sober thought. Obviously, her illness is very much alive even though it is presently kept under control with her medications.

As Linda contemplates her future state of health, she frequently meets others who have just experienced tick bites. Citing two new reports of tick exposure by her neighbors, she said, "On my way home, I gave my neighbor a ride, and he told me that he had bull's-eye rashes all over his back the day before yesterday. He went to the emergency room, and they gave him three weeks on antibiotics. I [also] took a tick off the 2-year-old across the street a couple of weeks ago." Worried over these incidences, Linda is concerned about her neighbors and how the disease will impact them in the coming years.

Advancing Vectors

Linda, who has continued to fight her battle on the front lines of Lyme disease in Connecticut, expressed her somber awareness that a certain subset of people with Lyme disease do not become *just* sick but chronically and painfully so with severe disabilities. Likewise, family members of the ill suffer their own real pains as they support and offer care to Lyme patients.

As the population of infected ticks has multiplied and spread into new territories, the number of families afflicted by Lyme disease and other tick-borne infections has increased correspondingly. When Linda first became infected, the ticks inhabited the grassy field across the road from her house. Fourteen years later, they now inhabit her front lawn as well. Understandably, the Rinaldi's have begun to look for a new home in town. In the meantime, their battle against tick invasion has not been as successful as they had hoped. Their pets have carried dozens of ticks into the house, ultimately infiltrating the Rinaldi's last place of refuge from these unwelcome vectors. Sadly, in 1999, their daughter, Bethany, also contracted Lyme disease.

Even with Linda's experience, months passed before her daughter's disease was properly diagnosed and a treatment protocol established. Bethany's illness was complicated by the presence of another tick-borne disease (co-infection), babesiosis, a malarial-like blood infection. "[Bethany] just about lost her last two years in high school, left dance, left cheerleading, and left volunteering at the hospital," recalled Linda. At this point in time, Bethany has recovered well and is essentially symptom-free except for some fatigue, occasional joint pain, and stamina limitations.

Fortunately, Linda's husband and son have not contracted any tick-borne infections. That has been a double blessing since both Linda and Bethany relied upon the help of healthy family members during their most severe periods of illness. "They have been very supportive [over] the years," Linda said.

Reflections

Linda's long journey to health was a roller coaster of hope and disappointments, of wise choices and some mistakes. In hindsight, it really should not have been as difficult as it was for Linda. After all, by the time Linda first contracted the illness, Lyme disease had been identified in Connecticut and recognized there for over a dozen years. Yet, oddly, the medical community in that state remained unaware of how to diagnose or treat it. Then too, limited thinking physicians made it difficult for Linda to fully explore any possible physical causes of her symptoms by rapidly concluding that her disease was probably psychiatric. As a result, the burden of medical research and advocacy fell on her own shoulders, bowed as they were from illness and frequent discouragement.

She also did not have the research advantages of the Internet as many have had since then. Still, she did what she could—she spoke openly about her illness with others, hoping that one of her listeners might know someone who could help her. Today, there are organized support groups, but Linda did not have that benefit when she needed it. Eventually, it was her own outspokenness that led her to a cooperative doctor who treated her with compassion and knowledge.

What she has learned from her experience may give other Lyme victims a valuable "heads up." She said, "The most important lesson I have learned from this experience was that people place too much faith in the medical community. If you happen to see 10 different doctors, you may get 10 different opinions. Go with your gut feeling and what seems right to you. Research, research, research...the information is out there if you just have access to the Internet."

Since Lyme disease symptoms may be similar to those of other diseases such as fibromyalgia, chronic fatigue syndrome, and multiple sclerosis, the disease can be easily misdiagnosed and overlooked by the medical community. Linda was correctly diagnosed because she focused on her "gut feeling," her faculty of self-awareness that bore witness to her whenever some medical advice seemed inappropriate.

The correct diagnosis finally led to ongoing treatment that has allowed Linda to function satisfactorily at work and at home. Antibiotics have kept her aggressive symptoms at bay. Understandably then, she is protective of the quality of life she possesses. "At this point on antibiotics, I can live a fairly decent life. I have symptoms and sometimes [I] really don't feel great, but it is very livable. Right now, I just want a life. I don't want to mess with the quality of life that I have now."

While she continues to guard her health and the lifestyle it permits her, she also remains vigilant for any medical announcements concerning new treatments for Lyme disease. As Linda patiently waits, she looks for the silver lining in what has been a long struggle for health. She stoically notes, "I see the world in a whole different light, [and] I feel as though I have the wisdom and knowledge of an elderly person. There are *some* positive things about going through a journey such as the one I have been through."

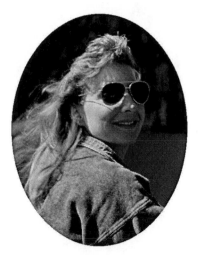

Danette

Northern Exposure

"Never ever give up!"
—*A Frog Fable*

In the vast wilderness of British Columbia, Canada, where the North and South Thompson Rivers merge, lies the city of Kamloops, Tournament Capital of British Columbia and home to 85,000 people.

The surrounding countryside provides a four season playground for locals and tourists. It is comprised of a wealth of lakes, streams, and the largest concentration of waterfalls in Canada. The grasslands and hills are dotted with a colorful spray of spring and summer wild flowers. The mountains are covered with dense forests of tall firs, cedars, and trembling aspens. Hidden deep within the forest interior or "bush," as the locals sometimes call it, thrives an abundance of wildlife:

eagles, bears, moose, songbirds, coyotes, wolves, mule deer, and cariboo among other creatures.

Forestry in the Kamloops area has surpassed ranching as the primary industry. With several mills in the area, loggers are kept busy in the bush, unless of course, their machinery breaks down. This was the case in the spring and summer of 1998 when some loggers called for an on-site repairman. The "man" that answered that call was a free-spirited, 34-year-old Kamloops woman named Danette "Dannie" MacDonald.

At five foot six inches, this blonde-haired valedictorian from the University College of the Cariboo in Kamloops was eager to don her coveralls and get her hands into the tool chest. She and her partner, Charlie, own and operate a heavy machinery maintenance service, and maintenance calls from loggers are a common occurrence for them. "Most of our customers are loggers out in the forests, and we usually do repairs right where the equipment breaks down," Danette explained.

Armed with insect repellent and her coveralls, she felt protected from most insects. "Generally I was only concerned about mosquito bites mainly because they're annoying. We usually had 'Deep Woods Off' on board the service truck, but unless the area was thick with mosquitoes—some places were really bad—we didn't bother. Depending on the time of year, I'd usually wear shorts, socks, runners, and a tank top underneath my coveralls. If I was there mainly for safety reasons—as it might be a one person job—I wouldn't bother putting on my coveralls, and I'd wander about the near surrounding area when I wasn't passing an occasional tool to Charlie," Danette said.

Sometime during that particular spring and summer when she worked in the bush, Danette noticed a red ring about two inches in diameter on her left forearm. It had a strange, tiny, black speck in the center of it. She recalled,

"It didn't hurt, and I thought maybe I had placed my arm up against the end of a hot tube or something a few days before, and now it was just a mark. Whatever. It went away after about a week, and I forgot about it." Danette enjoyed the rest of that summer and early fall in seemingly good health.

By October however, she started to experience a nagging backache with a headache and other flu-like symptoms that recurred off and on over the next two months. In fact, the symptoms never really went away, and she was puzzled because she rarely ever got sick.

Appeals for Help

The pain from her symptoms increased, and on December 15, a tearful Danette admitted herself into the emergency room of the local hospital complaining of acute back pain. The physician on duty asked, "Was there a pop or snapping sound?" He questioned her further about the level of stress she might have placed on her back from her physical work, thinking she had injured it somehow. Oddly, no x-rays were ordered, and the physician's diagnosis was inconclusive. He did, however, address her pain by prescribing Tylenol 3 and by recommending that she take time off from work to see a physiotherapist.

Without x-rays, the physiotherapist started Danette on an exercise program that was incredibly painful for her to perform. "The more I exercised, the worse it got. Instinct was telling me I was doing more damage than good, so I stopped going to her." Finally in February of 1999, Danette went to see her primary care physician. He prescribed more Tylenol 3 tablets which she used sparingly because of her borderline allergic reaction to codeine. He also referred her to a skilled massage therapist, but he could not relieve her of the painful symptoms either. Again, she had only prescription pain relievers to give her some measure of comfort.

She decided to also visit her trusted chiropractor whom she had seen for occasional spinal manipulations over the years. On one visit to this practitioner, Danette was told that "it" [the mysterious back pain] sometimes took up to two years for recovery. Danette naturally wondered, "Up to two years to recover from what?" No one had yet given this painful ailment a name.

Her pain was increasing, and sleep was nearly impossible. "I'd sleep for 20 minutes and wake up wishing I was dead, [then] change positions, fall asleep, [then again] wake up wishing I was dead, change positions...and I'd do this all through the night." Desperate for help, Danette tried to see her primary care physician again. He was not available, so she accepted an appointment with his clinic associate.

With a sense of starting all over, Danette related her medical history to this new doctor. After hearing her describe her various pains, he prescribed Demerol and referred her to another physiotherapist, his wife. "I was hoping that perhaps having them both as a team would work to my benefit," Danette thought.

Meanwhile, working as a mechanic became increasingly difficult even with Demerol. Sometimes when the medicine failed to mask her pain, she desperately resorted to combining her medication with a beer or two. "I would always do my best to wait as long as I could stand it before taking anything stronger than extra strength Tylenol or other over-the-counter pain pills. On a good day, I could go until 5 p.m. before having to give in to the narcotic-type drugs," Danette said.

Then a new symptom appeared, painful pressure in her ears. She returned to her doctor for some help when the pain finally became unbearable. "Before even looking at my ears, he told me all about how it's probably just a wax build-up," Danette recalled. He cautioned her about the improper use of certain ear cleaning products. She listened to his informative oration, and yet, he did not examine her ears. "I had to all but beg him to actually look at my ears, and after he examined them, he informed me that I did indeed have an infection in both ears."

Danette dutifully returned to the physiotherapist but found she felt even worse from the prescribed exercises. After doing what was asked of her, Danette said, "I was finding it necessary to use my pain killers more frequently." In addition to the pain, Danette noticed that she had been gaining weight. "I had gone from size three to five to a nine and had to buy bigger jeans throughout these progressions. Needless to say, I enjoyed the comments that came with this ...NOT!"

Physical Limitations Appear

Gradually, Danette realized that she could no longer work with Charlie as a mechanic. Still wanting to be of some help to him, she did a fair share of the business paperwork and ran errands. She struggled with sinking self-esteem and often felt "physically useless." Anxiety soon came in waves, and she thought it was due to her frustration over her physical limitations. However, she became very suspect of her condition when she also began feeling heart palpitations and sharp pains in her chest. Frightened, she thought perhaps she ought to quit smoking.

In addition to those new symptoms, she started to experience numbness, tingling, burning, and general aching in her legs. These worrisome sensations increased until, finally one morning, she woke up and could not feel anything in her lower left leg from the knee down. "You could have set fire to my pant leg, and I wouldn't have felt it," Danette recalled.

Fortunately, she had an appointment with her

physiotherapist that morning. After her examination, the concerned therapist scheduled an emergency appointment for Danette to see her physician husband. He, in turn, theorized that Danette might have pinched a nerve and then stated that if a person just shook the numb limb, the feeling would quickly return. Angered at the suggestion, Danette replied, "Yes, sometimes I find that [to be the case] too, but you may have noticed that I have never come in here for that [reason]!" Danette had experienced pinched nerves before, but in her mind, this was clearly something more serious than that.

Since the doctor did not appear very concerned, she asked to be referred to a neurologist. The doctor said that a neurologist probably couldn't do anything for her either, and he assured Danette that it wasn't like she would end up in a wheelchair or "anything like that." Completely disappointed, Danette left the examining room "feeling once again like I had been dismissed as just another hypochondriac."

As if Danette did not have enough symptoms to deal with, she also noticed that her menstrual cycles were becoming so painful that—for the first time—she contemplated relief through suicide. She returned to her primary care physician again for help. He prescribed some pain relievers, and when these did not work, he referred Danette to a gynecologist. The latter recommended a hysterectomy without an explanation.

This procedure was flatly rejected by Danette, and she returned to one of her former doctors. He recommended an injection of Depo-Provera, a form of birth control, which would be effective for three months. The theory behind this prescribed treatment was to regulate menstruation and cramping. Danette explained what happened over the next few months, "Talk about back-fire! Instead of getting any relief, my symptoms doubled!"

Danette went back to the physician who had prescribed this medication and asked him again to refer her to a neurologist. He responded that the referral paperwork process took a little time, and so she gave him two weeks. When she returned and discovered that he had not yet filled out the paper work, Danette reacted, "Totally stunned by this, I stood up and walked out the door without saying a word. [It was] my way of saying, 'You're fired!'"

The Passing of Time and Health

Eighteen months had passed since Danette's first flu-like symptoms had appeared, and still she lacked a diagnosis and, of course, a curative treatment plan. Struggling desperately, she now developed bladder control problems. "I could live with the fluctuating diarrhea and constipation—annoying as they were—but partially peeing my pants was not amusing to me at all." So back to the emergency room she went.

Once again, she retold her medical history to the emergency room physician. She recounted, "[First there was] the initial flu that turned into an incredible back pain that was comparable to intermediate back labor in child birth, the irritated bowel resulting in chronic diarrhea or constipation, the numbness, tingling, burning sensations that would migrate at any strength they desired in any area they wanted, the stomach aches, the weight gain (moved up to a size 12 now), and the embarrassment of bladder control problems that had now started."

While she took a breath to pause from her story, the doctor explained that, generally speaking, "We don't worry about this unless you have completely lost bladder control." With great restraint Danette replied, "Okay, let me see if I understand what you're saying. What you're telling me is that if I completely pee my pants that is a problem, but if I only partially pee my pants, that is acceptable?" After a long and uncomfortable stare-down, the physician suggested that perhaps she should consult with a neurologist. Danette's mind quietly whispered, "Good idea!"

At last, she had her long-awaited examination with a specialist in neurology. He began by questioning her, "After 18 months, you're complaining about this *now*?" Danette responded, "No, I have been complaining about this since it started, but I keep getting more hoops to jump through, and some of them are getting to be pretty repetitive! I can't get any help for some reason. Nobody seems to care, and I don't understand why!"

The neurologist ordered a CAT scan, and the results came back unremarkable. Consequently, he ordered an MRI, but the patient waiting list was nine months long. In the meantime, the specialist suggested that Danette lose some of those 30 extra pounds that she had gained. Easy for someone who overate, but Danette wasn't eating all that much, and exercise had proven very painful for her. Brought close to tears once again, Danette thought, "I'm not able to take much more of this minimizing of whatever is wrong with me! Doesn't anybody care enough to help me help myself? For [heaven's] sake, somebody please help me!"

Process of Elimination Begins

Since the wait for an MRI was so long, Danette wanted to be seen by another physician, albeit the sixth. In his examining room, she related her long story "in *Reader's Digest* style" to him. The doctor felt some empathy for her and promised to try, even if it took 50 attempts, to properly diagnose her condition. His sincere words were reassuring to her.

The next six months were filled with medical procedures of all kinds, including x-rays, a bone scan, and many other tests that Danette felt should be performed for a truly thorough clinical evaluation. In thinking about possible illnesses she might have, she recalled that the doctor she fired had suggested that she might have multiple sclerosis. A firm diagnosis for the disorder could not be established because she exhibited many symptoms that were not commonly associated with it.

Next, she was sent to a urologist, and he prescribed two popular analgesic drugs meant to relieve the symptoms of osteoarthritis, rheumatoid arthritis, as well as, pain from dysmenorrhea. Neither of these prescriptions did anything but drain her bank account.

By September 2000, Danette's stamina for walking had diminished greatly. She hesitantly resorted to the use of a wheelchair, especially for shopping. Remembering a trip to a local store, she said, "We needed to go to Costco to buy supplies for the shop and do some shopping for home stuff as well. I took a 50 mg tablet of Demerol 20 minutes in advance and filled my flask with alcohol so I could manage to sit in the truck." When she arrived at her destination, she reclined on the truck's bench seat for a while to stretch her back before stepping out into the parking lot. Trying to be helpful, Charlie grabbed a wheelchair and brought it up to her. "Tears formed and sat on the brim of my eyelids, but I was *not* going to cry. For the first half hour, I prayed to God that nobody I knew would see me, and I absolutely could not believe I had been reduced to this."

Inside the store, Danette's thoughts wandered to that place in her mind where humor is born. She whispered to her youngest daughter who was pushing her up and down the aisles, "The next time Charlie pushes my wheelchair, I am going to tilt my head sideways, let the drool drip out the side of my mouth, twitch and make severely handicapped sounds." Humor had often been Danette's coping mechanism, and it came to her rescue again that day at Costco in an otherwise humiliating situation.

Eventually, however, Danette did reach her breaking point and was hospitalized for a week. "After two years of being sent here and there, poked and prodded, taking test after test, I finally broke down crying uncontrollably." Her hard sobs were like those of a sobbing wife bent over the still body of her husband. Never before had the once confident and self-reliant Danette ever allowed herself to be seen crying, let alone like this. "I had reached the end of my rope, and I couldn't take it anymore," she said.

In the hospital, a neurosurgeon ordered a test for multiple sclerosis. The test results were negative, and the doctor subsequently ruled out this disease. Danette never saw him again. Frequently, the hospital staff questioned her about her "sciatic pain" and gave her heavy doses of pain relievers, which were greater than anything she had ever taken before. Danette was beginning to feel that her admission to the hospital was a lost cause.

When she saw a picture of polyps on the wall of the hospital ward, she wondered if her illness might be related to a growth pressing against her spine causing her excruciating pain. She questioned one physician about this possibility, and he told her that she ought to consult a gynecologist. *Great! Another hoop to jump through*, she thought.

Professional Judgment

During her hospital stay, Danette tried some gentle stretching exercises. "I felt like a very stiff 80-year-old woman all of the time. Even though I refused to give up, by now I was lucky if I could walk an entire city block. I couldn't even make one lap around the hospital ward I was in." She sat on the edge of her hospital bed and tried doing some simple leg exercises. A nurse saw her attempts and told Danette that this kind of exercise would be impossible to do if Danette really had a back problem, as she claimed.

Consequently, the nurse reported her observations to the doctor, and Danette, thereafter, was suspected of feigning illness for the purpose of satisfying a drug habit. The next morning, Danette was discharged, and her physician refused to prescribe any further pain relievers other than Tylenol 3. She was told that she was a strong person and was encouraged to exercise, and eventually everything would be okay.

In actuality, her physical condition spiraled downward quickly, and her disabilities became even more prominent. "The guilt of not being able to cook [for my family] was more than heartbreaking. Imagine that I can't walk. I can't cook a meal because the pots are too heavy, and I can't stand on my own two feet long enough to complete such a simple task, yet [I'm told], 'This is all in your head.'" By this time, Danette was having a productive day at home if she just washed, dried, and folded a single load of laundry.

Gynecological Discoveries

Though weak in body, Danette's mind was driven to find a label to this illness. "I hit the Internet to find out what was causing all this grief. I found an article on fibroids of the uterus. Everything matched!" She took that article with her when she saw her doctor again. He listened and thought it was a possibility. After two weeks of her persistence, he finally ordered testing and referred her to a gynecologist again.

When Danette saw this new doctor, she was experiencing break-through bleeding and severe nonstop uterine cramping. This specialist ordered a vaginal ultrasound, which for her was a very painful procedure. The results showed that she had multiple small fibroids with a possible adenomyosis (a painful disease of the uterine lining).

As a result, Danette had a hysterectomy on January 17, 2001. Surgery confirmed the presence of fibroids, adenomyosis, and revealed an ovarian cyst. Danette responded, "Right off the bat there was an instant improvement, and I was sure I had finally beat it. I could walk, stand and sit longer than before, and the pain had been literally cut in half."

Two weeks later she was back to work running small errands. She paced herself, conserving her energy to heal properly, yet plenty of symptoms remained. "I never completely recovered [after surgery]. The pain was less, but the numbness, tingling, and aching were returning slowly. Everything else, such as the bladder problems, bowel problems, dizziness, etc., stayed the same as before surgery."

Finally, Danette's long awaited MRI appointment came due. She underwent the procedure and waited for those results. She also had a colonoscopy to rule out colon disease. The colonoscopy showed a healthy colon, another reason for relief yet continued bewilderment for Danette. The MRI results came in and revealed a suspicious spot, so another MRI was scheduled a few months later. When the second set of images were viewed and read, the neurologist said that the suspicious spot had apparently disappeared.

"Too bad the symptoms didn't disappear with it," Danette said. In fact, Danette was now also suffering from vertigo and episodes of losing consciousness. She had not told the doctors this new information since she had just about lost her faith in them. "After all, it wasn't like they were going to take me seriously and do anything about it. I'm just a prescription druggie with imaginary problems, and I was back to fight for pain killers again."

She felt that she was back to square one, only now she was experiencing shortness of breath. Again she thought about ending her smoking habits. She developed night sweats so badly that she awoke dripping wet and had to change her sleep wear. Her hands and feet were always cold. "If I got cold to the bone, the pain would intensify, and it would take hours to warm up and days for the pain to simmer down," she explained.

Her expanding list of symptoms now included swelling of her hands and her legs from the knees down. She also experienced ringing in the ears and sensitivity to sharp, high-pitched sounds such as childrens' voices. Vision problems began to develop—irritating floaters and extreme light sensitivity. Though never diagnosed as dyslexic before, she now noticed that she reversed letters and numbers and found herself at the wrong places. She felt tired all the time, and her moods swung like a pendulum. She began to feel as if she was teetering on the brink of insanity. "Although I had good reasons to be depressed, such as being a prisoner of my now size 16, non-functional, self-torturing body, I wasn't depressed—just angry. I wanted my life back!"

Fibromyalgia?

Four years of painful suffering had passed since Danette's first symptoms, and she was learning new ways of being her own advocate. She never gave up searching for answers or requesting that this or that test be performed. She kept up her process of disease elimination whether or not she had a physician who believed in her. She considered fibromyalgia. "If indeed I had fibromyalgia, it was very important to quit smoking." Finally, on October 7, 2002, both she and Charlie stopped smoking.

Next she went to see a rheumatologist who ultimately diagnosed Danette with fibromyalgia. Danette was still not sold on this diagnosis, but "at that point, any answer was better than no answer," she reasoned. Danette began attending pain management meetings, and it was there that she became aware that her memory was giving out and that her concentration and comprehensive skills were nearly shot. She described it as "brain fog."

Connecting with the other patients at these meetings frightened her. "I became disgruntled with the idea that life would always be like this and there would be no cure. It upset me that I fit right in. Everything fit except for one thing, a nagging question in the back of my mind. If nobody knows what causes fibromyalgia, how do I know for sure that it's not something else? Gut instinct was telling me that somewhere I had missed the boat."

She searched the Internet and found an article by Dr. Gabe Mirkin about fibromyalgia. The first section in the article was "How to treat Lyme disease." Thinking this was a mistake, Danette dismissed the article and went to one that listed diseases sometimes mistaken for fibromyalgia. Among those conditions listed was Lyme disease.

Lyme Disease

With Mirkin's article in hand, she went to see her primary care physician again. Since her surgery, this doctor had once again become a more cooperative source of medical care for her. Together, they went through the list she found of conditions that mimic fibromyalgia and eliminated about 75% of them.

Tests were begun for the remaining 25% of the diseases that were listed in the article. The doctor ordered Western blot tests and an ELISA for Lyme disease through the provincial lab. "Everything was negative, negative, negative, and my heart was sinking until we came to the Lyme disease ELISA: Reactive!" Confidently, Danette's physician declared, "You have Lyme disease."

At this point, a flood of emotion came over Danette. Speechless, she could only point to a picture on the wall of the examining room showing a frog whose head was halfway down a crane's throat but whose arms were still desperately trying to strangle the throat of the crane. It read, "Never ever give up!" As she silently pointed to that struggling frog, tears streamed down her face. "After four years of incredible suffering, unable to work full time during the last three and a half of that, the emotional, mental, and psychological abuse I suffered from a majority of the medical professionals, I finally had an answer!"

Though her doctor had seemingly identified her illness at last, he honestly confessed that he knew very little about the complexities of, and treatment protocols for, Lyme disease. She appreciated his humble honesty and decided to find someone who was knowledgeable about the disorder. While still at the office, she quickly called Charlie with the news, and his reaction was "Thank God!" With sighs of relief, she and Charlie felt that perhaps an answer had been found.

Danette immediately took the test results to her rheumatologist. She expected him to be happy that her illness had finally been identified, but instead, he told her that females had a tendency to test falsely positive on the ELISA. He added that since her Western blots were negative for surveillance, he felt certain that Danette did not have Lyme disease. He added, "Besides, we do not have Lyme disease here. It's a good thing I did not give you antibiotics." The rheumatologist then recommended that she consult with an infectious disease specialist as a next step.

Utterly shocked at his quick dismissal of her test results, she agreed to see the physician he was recommending, but at the same time, she had a plan of her own. "I knew from my research that I should start on a minimum of 100 mg of doxycycline, twice daily, at the very least. In tears, I called my regular doctor's office and got in almost immediately." Her doctor could not understand the response she received from the rheumatologist and agreed to write a two month prescription for doxycycline to get her started on treatment.

The date was November 28, 2002, four years since Danette's suffering began. Meanwhile, Danette's newest challenge was to find a doctor who could confirm the Lyme diagnosis and recommend a treatment protocol.

Empowered by Knowledge

Again, the Internet became a helpful source in this search. Only two or three hours away from Kamloops, Danette found a physician who had experience treating Lyme disease. She got an appointment within days of calling. With her faithful mate, Charlie, they met with the new doctor. Her examination showed neurological and cognitive dysfunction, and her short term memory performance was poor. When asked to memorize three simple words for the duration of the exam, she could not do it. "Me, the valedictorian of 1991-92, could not remember three simple words. Me, the waitress that used to be able to take an order from a table of eight people without writing anything down and nail it every time...could not remember those three lousy words!" At the end of her thorough examination, the doctor stated that he was fairly confident that Danette had Lyme disease, but he also ordered additional blood tests to be done at a lab of his choice.

Knowing that Danette had been on doxycycline for three days, the doctor asked how she was feeling. She answered, "I had noticed that my hands, knees, and other joints had swollen up again but more so than it had before, and I was feeling achier than normal, plus I had a fairly good headache." He replied, "It could get worse, you know." He was speaking of the various Herxheimer-like reactions that Danette might experience when starting treatment. She wasn't completely aware of this element of the healing process, but she trusted her doctor. "I was so relieved to be finally listened to and understood," Danette said.

She and Charlie returned home with a feeling of satisfaction that Danette had finally set foot on the right path for the first time in four years. When she was home, she sat at her make-up dresser and wept. "I'm not sure if I was grieving all the lost time and suffering or if I was weeping relief that the hardest part of the battle was over. Perhaps I was mourning the way this disease had not only stolen my body from me, but it had also stolen a good part of my brain."

Treatment Reaction

Shortly thereafter, Danette felt the Herxheimer-like reaction in full force. "I ached so severely, and nothing helped me anymore. Having read [on the Internet] that it only lasts a few days, I hunkered down and sucked it up." Shortly after this, the results from the latest blood tests arrived and showed positive on the IgG and very closely positive on the IgM Western blot tests. With this information, she felt even more certain that the doctor's diagnosis was correct.

On December 28th, 2002, the physician started Danette on a treatment regimen using two antibiotics, Biaxin and tinidazole, both taken twice daily. After seven months on these antibiotics, Ceftin replaced the Biaxin. In February, Danette consulted with an infectious disease doctor. She was curious whether or not he would agree with the Lyme diagnosis she had received.

The physician was young and admitted that he had studied about Lyme disease five years ago. Danette explained that knowledge had advanced since then and that she was following Dr. Joseph Burrascano's November 2002 treatment guidelines. The doctor did not recognize his name or know of his studies in treating Lyme disease. However, Danette's insistence that Dr. Burrascano was a reputable and experienced Lyme disease physician may have been the reason he decided to document her current treatment regimen.

After doing so, he expressed his opinion that any antibiotic treatment extending longer than three months was reckless, and that as a patient, Danette was taking unnecessary risks. He informed Danette that he would be sending reports to three of her recently seen physicians stating that she *may have had* Lyme disease, and if that was the case, she was now cured because she had received "enough" antibiotic.

Rapid Improvement

Despite the young doctor's disapproval, Danette continued on extended antibiotic treatment, and her symptoms began to abate. Six months into Danette's treatment, she was able to travel on holiday. "I'm proud to be able to boast of the fact that I could do all of the driving, all of the cooking and cleaning, chop small amounts of firewood; and when Charlie asked if he could help, my answer was 'Yes, go hold down the picnic table with this beer for me, will ya please?' I was beginning to have a life again!"

Danette's treatment had extended beyond 17 months, and during that time, the regimen was modified at intervals to meet her needs. In January 2004, her medications were adjusted from Ceftin to Biaxin XL, twice daily, and taken concurrently with tinidazole. This treatment seemed to work well for Danette, since she gained back the greater percentage of her health. "I might not ever reach 100%, but that's okay because I have most of my life back again, and for that, I am more than grateful. I feel like one of those second chancers, and as a result, I stop to smell the roses now, and they are beautiful!"

A Voice in the Wilderness

Danette's advice to those who have symptoms like fibromyalgia—or have been diagnosed with fibromyalgia—is straightforward. "I can't stress enough how important it is to be your own advocate by seeking answers for yourself, by double checking that diagnosis with all the information available to you." In her search for answers, Danette outspokenly shared her medical information with anyone who would listen. "I was talking to everyone I knew about my symptoms and how it was affecting me. As a result, a good neighbor and friend suggested that maybe it was fibromyalgia, [the key] which, in turn, led me to the correct diagnosis of Lyme disease."

Her own voice which had been crying out—as it was—alone in the wilderness, had finally been heard and constructively answered. She won the greatest battle of her life by never giving up and, more importantly, by one other means. "I listened to my body. Wasn't that what all of these doctors were supposed to do?" she asked. Danette MacDonald had reason to be angry at the failures of the medical professionals who examined her over the course of four years, but she explained, "Instead of harboring an unhealthy anger, I now devote my spare time to sharing what I know with others. If by sharing my hard-learned education about Lyme disease with others changes just one life for the better, I've accomplished something."

However, Danette does not end with this point. "There's nothing I wish more than to be able to educate as many physicians and patients as I can by using my own case as living proof that Lyme disease does exist here [in British Columbia] and that long-term antibiotic therapy does work."

Postscript

In November 2004, Danette was taken off her antibiotic therapy, and she continued to maintain good health. By March 2005, she reported, "I'm doing pretty good! Into my fifth month [off] antibiotics, still doing lots of detox and supplements, and still training at kickboxing and Chinese Gung Fu. This March 28th, I'm getting married to Charlie, so life is a bit busy, but it's all coming along very well."

For Danette (MacDonald) Cade, her recovery from Lyme disease was a long journey. She reached a measure of health that she considers a success story, and she credits her strong relationship with Charlie for part of that success. For the past seven years, he's been her loyal advocate and caregiver. He's seen her through some pretty tough times. Appreciatively, she said, "Charlie is one of those guys that makes you wanna throw rocks at the rest. I'm not sure I would have made it through all this if he hadn't been here in all the ways he was with me."

After one year of being off all antibiotics, Danette reported that she was still enjoying good health. She said, "I'm still doing great, and [I] am ready now for my yellow belt...Whoo hoo!" Finally, life is sweet again, and she's not wasting a minute of it.

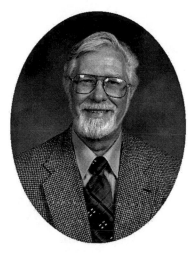

Glenroy

Thorn in the Flesh

"For when I am weak, then I am powerful."
—*II Corinthians*

As a New Hampshire farm boy, Glenroy Wolfsen enjoyed all the healthful pleasures of country living. Nourished on farm fresh produce from the family garden and creamy, rich cow's milk, Glenroy never knew serious illness during his youth. Instead, he was a happy and musically gifted child, and he eventually polished those talents at Westminster Choir College in Princeton, New Jersey. From there, he attended Trenton State College for Musicology and then followed his spiritual quest at New Brunswick Theological Seminary for a Master of Divinity degree.

He worked actively as a pastor and as a church and synagogue musician, enjoying to the full his physical and mental health. He thought of himself as "a well-rounded person with no health problems at all" until he contracted Lyme disease at about 57 years of age. His earlier adult life was pleasantly routine when, in 1964, he met and married his wife, Patricia, who shared many of the same passions with him. They resided in High Bridge, Hunterdon County, New Jersey, where they both taught music in the public schools and raised their four children, three daughters and one son.

When Glenroy was about 49 years old, Patricia was diagnosed with multiple sclerosis, while at the same time, his daughter was undergoing kidney dialysis. He left his job to take care of his daughter until her premature death in 1992 and later, when Patricia was no longer able to teach, he also became her home caregiver.

First Symptoms

In June of 1998, Glenroy noticed feeling a little more fatigued than normal, especially when exerting himself physically in necessary yard duties. He began experiencing very rapid heart beats in the afternoons with occasional irregular rhythms. He went to his family doctor who suspected that he was feeling the stress of caregiving and suggested that he relax more and drink an occasional glass of wine. Glenroy went home and followed his doctor's suggestions, but his symptoms persisted. Not only did they persist, but additional frightening symptoms began to appear.

"These [symptoms] began as odd sensations while driving the car with a bit of disorientation and sometimes not knowing the familiar roads I was traveling on," Glenroy recalled. Sometimes while parked, he felt utterly lost. Other times, when the vehicle was moving, he felt motion sickness. When cars sped past his vehicle, he felt he was going backwards. Glenroy noted, "I lost a sense of direction-orientation and compass points."

He also complained of feeling cold and shaky for

no apparent reason. His mental abilities became unusually dulled, and he felt that he perceived reality only from within the "cage" of his mind. These troubling conditions continued unabated from July until September of 1998. Anxiety over his sudden and alarming change of health added an additional burden upon an already taxed body.

These symptoms were, in fact, not the first signs of Glenroy's Lyme disease. "As I look back now, it seems to me that I can remember other incidents of isolated times when I was aware that I had a generalized strange sensation in my head that made normal tasks and driving feel very strange," he remembered.

A Pharmacist's Advice

One day, Glenroy went to his pharmacist to get supplies for his wife's care, and he described what he was personally going through: the fatigue, the heart problems, the heightened overall anxiety, the surfacing of panic attacks, tinnitus (ringing in the ears), and the odd brain sensations. "It was fortunate for me that he recognized my symptoms right away—he and his wife and two children all had Lyme disease at that time and were being treated as a family."

The pharmacist recommended that Glenroy see a doctor he knew in Pennsylvania, which he did in the fall of 1998. At that visit, blood samples were drawn and sent to a lab for analysis. The blood lab report indicated positive readings for Lyme disease, babesiosis (a malarial-like tick-borne infection), and ehrlichiosis (another tick-borne disease). At last, Glenroy knew what was causing his puzzling but rapid decline in health. The doctor quickly prescribed a treatment regimen for Lyme disease and the co-infections, and also, had Glenroy take some helpful dietary supplements.

At the onset of treatment, Glenroy noticed an increase

in his symptoms that included muscle spasms, cramping, and some loss of vision. His tinnitus worsened, and he noticed some loss of hearing in his left ear. Again, his heart exhibited rapid beating and irregular rhythms. He complained of increased fatigue, more difficulty driving, further panic attacks, and enhanced and seemingly unprovoked anxiety.

My Brother's Keeper

Meanwhile, Glenroy struggled to care for his wife whose multiple sclerosis was progressing. There were mornings when he could barely get out of bed; and yet because his wife depended upon his help, he pressed himself into painful movement. "This kept me moving when otherwise I am sure I would have stayed in bed," he said. Besides his wife, he had another person to think about.

Glenroy's teenage son, Michael, who suffered from choroideremia (an inherited eye disease that causes progressive loss of vision), was also living at home. With diminished vision, he watched on with all the anticipatory grief that one experiences when seeing a loved one gradually slip away. Glenroy said, "It was hard for him to see his mother going downhill each day. I did my best to care for him and cook the food and do all the other household duties necessary, as well as to give him attention and time and look out for his school work. I felt sometimes that all this involvement made it very difficult for me."

Source of Comfort

Glenroy sought comfort and peace by reading psychospiritual literature. "I read even if my brain-mind was not particularly understanding, which sometimes happened more than other times. I knew this was helping me keep my mental processes working, and it was also nourishing my mind and spirit." Glenroy felt particularly indebted to the writings of George I. Gurdjieff and his pupils, the journals of Jane Heap, and Maurice Nicoll's *Psychological Commentaries*. Glenroy examined Nicoll's two books on the parables and miracles of Jesus which gave him great insight into Jesus' power and work.

The resulting psychospiritual conclusions that Glenroy drew gave him solace while he struggled with his own personal "thorn in the flesh." "I learned that my fears, my anxieties, my self-pity, my anger, and hostility were not my real self. This was the disease and not my essence which was still untouched."

Helped by this analysis, he became more objective to his negative psychological states, and in that way, he preserved precious energy for healing. He also came to realize that if one practices the truth, "one is not alone even when lonely or abandoned, but that help from high powers is available through humility and asking, that is, by doing all that one is able to do and then turning problems over to that which is beyond oneself."

Another source of Glenroy's comfort and peace was his son, Michael, who encouraged him to return to his early love of writing poetry. He began to write a couple of poems each day in spite of his debilitating symptoms. "To my surprise and delight, while writing, there was a part of me that could create when my thinking-mind was not working well. I also found that when creating, my symptoms were not a part of my experience, or if they were, they became a part of the poetry."

This creative discipline gave Glenroy the intuition that he was not worthless and good-for-nothing and that, perhaps, something he wrote might be of value to others who were suffering from a similar "thorn in the flesh." Perhaps such individuals would see in his work a mind and heart that still had something to say when his body and brain were struggling with Lyme.

Valley of Deep Shadow

For three and one half years, Glenroy continued on treatment prescribed by his doctor. He noted some small improvement, but his heart troubles continued. At this point, his family members thought it would be better if Michael went to live with one of his sisters, in light of his mother's condition and Glenroy's inability to properly care for him. "I missed him a lot but tried to understand that they felt this was in his best interests. My wife's condition continued to deteriorate, and I was doing more for her because of the dangers inherent in her condition."

Furthermore, the family thought that because no significant progress had been made in the last three and one half years, Glenroy should consider switching to an alternative approach that was successful for other Lyme patients they knew.

Skeptical and afraid to leave his doctor, Glenroy hesitantly agreed to see the alternative doctor his family now recommended. This doctor individualized Glenroy's diet and treatment protocols and started him on a homeopathic remedy, supplements, and herbal formulations. Glenroy's diet mainly consisted of live foods, meaning foods that are uncooked and fresh including vegetables, fruits, soy products, and other unprocessed edibles. These foods are rich in nutrients and live enzymes and are thought to provide support to the immune and other body systems needed for healing to occur.

During the first two months of this transition from Western medical treatment to alternative therapy, an unexpected upheaval of Glenroy's symptoms ensued. "The head fog, disorientation, problems walking, paranoia, and anxiety levels were difficult to deal with," he recalled.

During this trying physical period, his wife, Patricia, was transferred from their home to a care facility, and then, to their daughter's home. Soon afterward, she died while under the merciful supervision of hospice care.

Remembering that day, Glenroy said, "I was so sick that I went to spend my own private time with her. I could not endure going to a public funeral." He also declined attendance at the burial because the trip was more than he could manage. Afterwards, in his acute grief, he felt quite alone in his home with only his dog as his companion. In spite of his sorrow and the daily realities of Patricia's absence, he remained determined to stay focused on carrying through with his new therapy to the best of his ability.

Once again, he drew solace from his books. "Although reading was more difficult, the books I had been studying were my constant companions." Even when he drove his car, Glenroy took a book along in case he felt like just getting out and sitting in a park for a while. Time passed in this fashion, and with each monthly visit to his doctor, his therapy regimen was adjusted to meet his changing needs.

Rebirth

Within a few months, Glenroy noticed some improvements, first physically and then cognitively. The ringing in his ears waned, and gradually, so did the anxiety and paranoia. He began to walk farther distances with time and felt cautious optimism. His creative juices returned to him, and he began to write again and to read with greater comprehension.

Most encouraging to Glenroy was his social rebirth. "I became more able to interact socially with other people and took more of an interest in helping other people I knew who were suffering with Lyme and co-infections." Most importantly, he was also ready to reunite with Michael. At that point in time, Glenroy had sold his home and moved to an apartment. It represented a new beginning for him, and he was excited to have Michael's companionship there.

Glenroy had endured the many unexpected and unwelcome changes in his life with humility and grace. He had come to know weakness and how it could empower him spiritually and psychologically.

Today, he has regained about ninety percent of his former good health. He continues to maintain that health through a good diet and an exercise program. Perhaps most profoundly, he has acquired a new attitude toward life—seeing it through eyes of greater understanding.

Having learned a wealth of lessons about himself during his illness, Glenroy remains gratefully enriched. He even restored some measure of the familiar back into his life. "I have gone back to part-time school teaching, playing the piano from time to time, attending church, and singing in the choir, and I'm working on getting some of my poetry published."

Glenroy's story does not end without this postscript, that he considers a special blessing from God. "I have met— first on the Lyme email group, then on the phone, and finally in person—a wonderful woman and fellow Lyme patient. She has brought love into my life, and more than that, we are helping to love, touch, nourish, and heal each other."

For Glenroy, it was a providential meeting and surely the climax to a courageous effort in his fight against Lyme disease. "I know that my suffering has had its blessings and its lessons; and most of all, an opportunity to live with a new purpose and a companion whose love has given me new life." Some silver linings just don't get any better than that.

ROSE
12/02/2002
by Glenroy Wolfsen

All around
Is frozen, cold and still,
Gray with black rocks
Rising behind the river.

Set on wooden posts
The black mailbox
And beside it
One red rose atop its stem.

Lifeless but holding
The blush of color,
The folds of a vibrant beauty.

There against the chill
It lifts a promise
Like the hope faith lifts
Against despair.

HANDS
11/08/2002
by Glenroy Wolfsen

I almost missed them in passing by.
It was a green field down from the park.

There, a small white bench with grass-green arm rests
And nestled in between
An old couple
With white hair
Sat together in the sun.

Sun rising on their sunset,
They sat
Holding hands
Holding in those hands
A life together lived
Holding yet memories,
So many things
Only they can know together

Holding what so many others
Have had to let go.

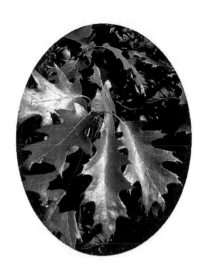

Raleigh Oaks

"Although the world is full of suffering,
it is also full of the overcoming of it."
—*Helen Keller*

Some years hold significant memories—perhaps a baby's first steps or a much needed vacation getaway for two. For 32-year-old *Christie Smith* and her husband, *Greg*, of Raleigh, North Carolina, the year 2002 was all of that and more.

Christie was the busy mother of two young boys. The eldest was three years old, and the youngest had just turned one that March. Besides raising the children, she also worked part-time as a graphics designer and writer. Between her responsibilities at home and at work, life was hectic. That is why Christie was really looking forward to getting away with Greg for a weekend in late April to celebrate their seventh wedding anniversary. Cabin quarters were already reserved at a century-old bed and breakfast high in the Blue Ridge Mountains of western North Carolina.

This relaxing weekend could come none too soon for Christie. Ever since her son was born, she noticed that she frequently felt moody. "I attributed a lot of that to [my] hormonal adjustment post delivery, although I felt it sure was taking a long time to even out. I felt tired a lot, but I was working part time and chasing a three year old, and I had a baby that didn't sleep through the night consistently." She just thought she needed a little time away from the demands of motherhood and her job.

Their vacation was everything they had hoped for— a leisurely afternoon sipping beers, lounging on deck chairs overlooking a pond, and watching a glorious sunset descend behind the silhouette of the trees in the distance. After dinner, they took a slow walk around the grounds. Then they retired to their quarters in a cozy cabin lit only by the amber glow of the gas stove inside. Outside, only the muffled sounds of the nocturnal critters could be heard. It was the perfect ending to a relaxing day.

The following morning was pleasantly warm. Christie recalled dressing in shorts and a sleeveless top and preparing for a morning hike before heading home later that day. After driving to a nearby mountain trail, she and Greg hiked for 45 minutes until the trail ended near a cold mountain stream. "It was a pleasant day," Christie remembered. What she didn't realize then was that it was one of the last pleasant days she would enjoy for a long time.

Home and Job

There's nothing like a little trip away to make home seem so appealing again. The Smith home was located in a neighborhood in Raleigh that was developed in the 1970s.

"[It] has an abundance of full grown trees, mostly oaks in our yard. Our lot was particularly woody with lots of natural areas because we could not get grass to grow in the [shady] back yard," Christie explained.

Within walking distance from their home was a pool and a park where Christie walked with the boys and their family dog, *Casey*, an eight-year-old golden retriever. Also within walking distance was a man-made lake. Christie said, "It had a great walking and running trail around the perimeter, and [I took] the boys and the dog there often to walk, fish, and ride bikes. We were an active family."

Christie was always very conscious of her health, and whenever possible, she opted for the more natural methods of health management. She gave birth to both of her sons without anesthesia and breast fed both boys for the first nine months of their lives. She refrained from taking prescription drugs, including birth control pills, and kept a very limited number of over-the-counter medications in the house. Christie said, "I [was] a healthy eater, subscribed to *Cooking Light,* and [even] bought some organic [foods]. My husband and I belonged to a gym where I had begun strength training with weights for the first time in my life, and [I] was really enjoying the results."

In addition to her home life, Christie also worked twenty to thirty hours a week as a graphics designer, writer, and editor. After returning from her weekend vacation, she jumped right back into the mainstream flow of work and demanding deadline schedules. Her immediate assignment was to produce a centennial history publication for her company. This work involved researching and writing the company's history and supervising its design layout and printing. The publication was needed for a centennial celebration at the end of May 2002, which gave Christie less than a month to produce it. "I was under a lot of stress at the time," Christie recalled.

Despite the pressures of this assignment and her frequent moodiness, she still felt capable of performing all that was expected of her. She reasoned that her moodiness was not uncommon for a post delivery mother. After all, she knew that postpartum adjustment can take as long as one year. By May 2002, it had been a full 13 months since her son's birth and four months since she weaned him from the breast. Despite the generous passage of time, Christie persisted in thinking that her hormones were still readjusting, although admittedly, she wondered why it was taking so long. She also acknowledged that she felt constant fatigue, but again she reasoned—with a three year old boy to chase after and with a baby who was not sleeping through the nights consistently—it was not unusual to be tired.

Escalating Symptoms

However, in mid-May, Christie did notice something unusual—pain and stiffness in her neck and left shoulder. Again, she dismissed these symptoms as merely stress induced aches and pains, nothing a good massage couldn't relieve. By early June, though, the pain still persisted and then began to escalate so that even her night's sleep became regularly disrupted. As a result, she consulted with her primary care doctor, and he diagnosed her condition as "a pinched nerve." He prescribed naproxen, a nonsteroidal anti-inflammatory drug (NSAID) that is used to relieve pain, inflammation, and stiffness in a number of conditions.

"Within a week of taking these medications, I began experiencing pain and tingling in my left arm and down into my fingers," recalled Christie. She immediately returned to her primary care doctor for a follow-up consultation, at which time x-rays were taken and an MRI of her cervical spine was done. Her doctor then referred her to a neurosurgeon for a possible problem with her cervical vertebrae.

While waiting for that appointment, Christie went in for her annual gynecological exam. She asked the physician's medical assistant whether or not it was normal for her to still be experiencing moodiness and fatigue more than a year after giving birth. The medical assistant responded by asking Christie if she wanted a prescription for an antidepressant. She answered, "I really don't feel comfortable taking something like that." Instead, Christie settled for a multivitamin and hoped that would take care of the matter.

Grin and Bear it

When Christie finally met with the neurosurgeon, he reviewed her earlier MRI films and determined that she had a cervical disc herniation. However, in his opinion, it was so minor that he did not recommend surgery. Instead, he arranged for Christie to undergo physical therapy, which she faithfully did for the next six weeks.

Rather than improving, though, Christie faced additional and alarming symptoms by August. She quickly returned to the neurosurgeon with complaints of new pains in her left leg in addition to the persisting pains in her neck and left shoulder area. "The neurosurgeon told me that he believed the two [pain sites] were unrelated and that people lived with aches and pains all the time."

His chin-up lecture fell upon shocked ears. Christie could not believe that he was telling her that things were tough all over and that she should just grin and bear it. She was summarily dismissed without further help or encouragement. Her immediate feelings of disgust and abandonment developed into confusion about which way to turn. In frustration, she quit all physical therapy since it was not helping her conditions improve. In fact, she had discontinued all exercise, and uncharacteristically—for her—started taking muscle relaxants daily and sleeping on a heating pad. Meanwhile, she was experiencing an increase in fatigue and moodiness, not to mention another new symptom, difficulty concentrating. "I felt my life was falling apart," Christie said.

Neurologist

In September, Christie consulted a neurologist. A battery of tests was run, including an MRI of her brain, blood arterial tests, and two nerve conduction tests. When the films were viewed and the other test results came in, the doctor reported to Christie that she was healthy by all test accounts. Still, a nagging doubt persisted in his mind. He knew that he had failed at diagnosing her ailment. In order to help resolve this diagnostic dilemma, he asked her to come back for another MRI in six months. Perhaps by then, something would appear that would lead to a diagnosis.

By October, the symptoms in Christie's left arm and leg had worsened to the point that her daily routine was nearly impossible. This once active woman of two youngsters was now easily exhausted from walking a block to the park with the boys. Even more sedate tasks, such as writing checks to pay the bills, made her affected arm feel like dead weight hanging from her shoulder.

Almost without exception, her fatigued limbs began to tighten involuntarily with painful muscle spasms. Despite all of her debilitating symptoms, Christie tried to perform her duties caring for the boys at home. She could barely wait for the moment when her husband walked through the door at the end of his work day. At that moment, the boys became Greg's instant charge as Christie retreated to her bed wracked with pain, exhaustion, and now—growing depression.

A Friend's Suggestion

One of Christie's friends, who was an oncologist, recommended that she see a different primary care physician. Christie willingly followed her friend's advice. At the appointment, the doctor asked Christie, "[Has] anyone run blood tests to rule out arthritis, chronic fatigue [syndrome], lupus, thyroid dysfunction, and Lyme disease?" She responded, "No." To actually try and find out what was at the root of Christie's situation, the physician ran a battery of tests that might suggest or rule out some of these possibilities. The results of those tests were surprising. "The only positive [indicator] out of the group was the Lyme disease titer," said Christie.

The doctor immediately prescribed a three-week course of doxycycline, and within the first few days, Christie noticed changes in her health. "At first my fatigue increased, but I began to feel better within a few days. It was so great to have energy again, to want to play with my kids, and to sleep without pain meds or a heating pad!"

During her antibiotic treatment, Christie continued to show improvement; however, one and a half weeks after her treatment ended, she began to feel ill again. Her former symptoms returned. Obviously, this short-term therapy was insufficient to be curative for Christie's case of Lyme disease.

She returned to her doctor for a follow-up exam. He could observe that despite finishing the recommended antibiotic treatment, his patient had not reached a state of recovery. Apparently, though, the doctor did not question whether the recommended three-week course of antibiotics was curative for Lyme disease. He did not seem to wonder why or act on the observation that improvement occurred with doxycycline therapy and was reversed when the drug was withdrawn. Perhaps, too, her persisting conditions caused him to doubt the correctness of his Lyme diagnosis. In any case, he again prescribed naproxen to somehow discern if her debilitating symptoms were caused by something other than Lyme disease.

After two days of this medicine, Christie's health plummeted. New symptoms appeared including ringing in her ears, insomnia, paralysis of the left side of her face (Bell's Palsy), as well as all of the earlier symptoms that began appearing since May. Her rapid deterioration and the astonishing number and type of symptoms that surfaced—especially the neurological presentations—were extraordinarily frightening to Christie, and she felt desperate to find someone who could help her. Time was truly of the essence.

An Internet Connection

It was now January 2003, seven months after the first symptoms had appeared in Christie's neck and shoulder. Desperate for some knowledgeable help, she went online to search for information about treating Lyme disease. She found the Lyme Disease Network website, and it ultimately led her to a knowledgeable doctor in her area. "Due to weather delays, I did not actually meet with the physician until March 2003. Until that time, my primary care doctor was kind enough to prescribe doxycycline for me," Christie explained.

At her appointment with the new physician, blood samples were taken in order to perform the necessary Western blot tests. The test results revealed that several key bands specific for the Lyme spirochete were positive. The doctor used the information from the test results in the context of a thorough medical evaluation and ultimately made a clinical diagnosis of Lyme disease. He suggested an intravenous therapy, but since Christie had the two small boys to care for, she decided that she would prefer oral antibiotic treatment instead. She began aggressive antibiotic therapy in early March, and for the next nine months, she continued a regimen of switching between four different antibiotics and other medications.

"I was well informed of the possible risks and side effects associated with this treatment, and I was tested regularly to make sure that my body was functioning normally while on this therapy," Christie explained. Over the next nine months, four antibiotics were employed: Biaxin, doxycycline, Cipro, and Augmentin. These antibiotics were rotated over time, and at night, Christie took 300 mg of Neurontin for her neck and arm nerve pain. Every now and then, the doctor prescribed a break, what Christie called her "holiday" from the rotation protocol. Then, every fourth week for seven days, another antibiotic, Flagyl, was introduced.

Whenever Christie took the seven day course of Flagyl, she experienced a temporary worsening of symptoms. "Over time, these [flare-ups] began to dissipate, and I began to feel better on my holidays off meds," she said.

Since aggressive antibiotic therapy can strain different systems of the body, supportive supplements such as a multivitamin, vitamin B6, and a high quality acidophilus were also added to her regimen. In addition, she learned that her occasional social smoking and alcohol consumption greatly intensified her Lyme disease symptoms, so she quit those behaviors in order to cooperate fully with her recovery plan.

After Therapy

In November, Christie finished the prescribed oral antibiotic therapy. "I took a leap of faith and stopped taking meds," she said. Christie concentrated immediately on rebuilding her immune system through dietary supplements and other natural methods.

She also incorporated yoga exercises back into her daily routine along with a weekly walking and swimming routine. "My energy is back; my mood is up. I feel like I've rediscovered an old friend," said Christie. When she does overexert herself, symptoms in her left leg, arm, and neck will flare. For this, she still takes Neurontin at night to relieve some of the nerve pain still present.

During the daytime, her pain and muscle weakness present difficulties on the job. "It is especially hard to write for extended periods of time. I am left-handed, and the strength in the left side of my body is still much less than on the right side," she said. Monthly visits to her family chiropractor help relieve some of the physical symptoms of affected limbs. Acknowledging the residual effects of her illness, Christie said, "I'm not sure that my battle is completely over, but I am worlds better than I was when I was first diagnosed."

Despite this, she knows that she has a safety net of sorts—two supportive and caring physicians in North Carolina who have the knowledge and skill to treat this complex disease. Without their help, she knows she would still be very ill today. Reflecting upon what her doctors did that made a difference, she said, "[My doctors] trusted me and what I was telling them. [They] are doctors who went beyond the norm to bring me back to a healthy and normal lifestyle."

After personally experiencing how quickly debilitating neurological involvement can occur in the progression of Lyme disease, Christie emphatically said, "Lyme disease ruins lives. I am one of the lucky ones. I know that now."

The Eternal How

Christie knew virtually nothing about Lyme disease in October 2002 when her doctor asked her if she spent a lot of time outdoors. She admittedly remembered having done a lot of camping, hiking, and cross country skiing across the United States and in Europe. However, it was impossible for her to pinpoint the place or event that led to her infection. She never noticed an attached tick or an erythema migrans rash, which appears—arguably—in about half of all cases. She also did not present with any super flu-like symptoms, as many do. She did not have any of these significant diagnostic indicators, which delayed a correct diagnosis in her case.

For these reasons, Christie will always wonder how and where she contracted the infection. "It is highly possible that I have had Lyme disease for many years, and it was latent until a stress, such as the birth of my second child or a stressful time at work, brought it out into my system." Stress has been shown to have a significant impact on suppression of the immune system in a number of studied disorders including infections, so this contention weights merit. While the resurgence of latent viral disorders following stressful conditions is well known, the complex interplay between disease, immune function, and stress is far from being fully understood.

A Canine Postscript

As much as the family recreated outdoors, no other family member contracted Lyme disease. However, in June 2004, the family's dog, Casey, did receive a diagnosis of Lyme disease. When Casey's vet ran the annual heart worm screening, which also screens for Lyme disease, it came back positive for Lyme. Consequently, the vet drew a sample of Casey's blood for further testing, and the results showed highly elevated levels of Lyme disease antibodies. The vet then prescribed a treatment for Casey—300 mg of doxycycline daily for three weeks.

This diagnosis was initially surprising to Christie because "for most of [Casey's] life, she had been on the medication that is supposed to deter fleas and ticks." After thinking about it longer, Christie realized that "I had gotten slack and was only applying [Casey's medication] in the summer and fall (six months) and not spring or winter."

Casey's diagnosis seemed to answer a lot of questions regarding her behavior over the previous six months. "Since October 2003, Casey was showing signs of fatigue and joint pain (stiffness upon rising and lying down). She was also losing a lot of hair for that time of year. Around December, she became noticeably edgy and nervous especially around neighborhood kids. She even began snapping at some of the kids, and we had to put her in a closed room when friends came over to play for fear of her hurting someone." At the time, the family attributed Casey's uncharacteristic behavior to old age aches and pains, but it was nothing of the sort.

The vet asked Christie if Casey had "been up north recently," but she had not. In fact, Christie said, "Casey had been in my home and [in the] back yard in Raleigh, North Carolina, for the last 12 months." Yes, Casey had been home, at Raleigh Oaks, and so the questions resurface. Was Christie also exposed and infected by ticks in her own thickly wooded back yard? Why not? As Christie said, "Ticks travel. Lyme disease is [nearly] everywhere." A simple check of CDC surveillance tables (easily done from any computer) or contact with the Department of Health reveals that the disease *does exist* in North Carolina. The risk is lower than in the Northeast, but it cannot be discounted by anyone who deals with human or animal disease.

Another consideration in Christie's case was the

oak trees in her back yard. Acorns are a favorite food for white-footed mice and white-tailed deer, two hosts for Lyme disease. Acorn production has been hypothesized to correlate positively with Lyme disease occurrence on the East Coast. While this hypothesis has not been fully substantiated—the ecological impact may be more complex than originally thought—one thing is certain, that the hosts for Lyme disease do live where acorns abound.

As for Casey, three weeks of doxycycline brought blessed relief from her Lyme disease symptoms, and she was back to her old self. However, after a month off medication, she began relapsing in a pattern so familiar to Christie. The vet was also reluctant to prescribe further antibiotics. When Casey was finally put back on the medication, her symptoms started to resolve again. The so called "curative treatment" failed once again. Christie had to question authority once again to obtain reasonable and logical therapy, but this time, Christie was not at all surprised.

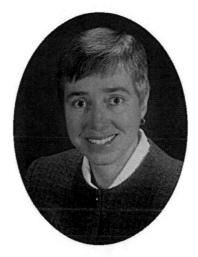

Joan

To Leave a Legacy

"To call myself beloved,
to feel myself beloved on earth."
—*Raymond Carver*

It seems to be the natural course of psychological inquiry to wonder about existence and self. Who am I? What is my purpose in life? What legacy will I leave to the next generation?

Joan McComas, Ph.D., of Kanata, Ontario, Canada, felt confident that she knew those answers. After all, she persevered over two decades to build an academic identity and profession. Initially, she earned her Bachelor of Science from McGill University in Montreal in 1970. A few years later, she married and moved to New Zealand where she became mother to three children, a daughter, born in 1975, and two sons born in 1977 and 1979. As she raised her children, she attended the University of Auckland where she earned a Masters of Science (1982) and a Ph.D. (1990), both in Psychology.

Immediately afterward, Joan accepted a position at the University of Ottawa as assistant professor. Five years later, after receiving her tenure, she was promoted to the post of director of the Physical Therapy program. Her achievements did not end there. Two years later, she was honored to become associate dean and director of the School of Rehabilitation Sciences.

As such, she was responsible for a teaching staff of 24 university professors and eight support staff. Under her care were more than 500 students in both undergraduate and graduate degree programs. She had supervisory responsibilities over an active rehabilitation research program that later brought her international recognition. She also promoted rehabilitation research and teaching as a member of various provincial and national committees.

On a community level, her contributions were numerous. She volunteered on administrative boards, reviewed grants, programs, and academic papers. She became a published scholar on the subject of rehabilitation and won grants to fund research. For Joan, climbing the academic ladder and enjoying its associated privileges was the result of purposeful planning and determination. "I have always known where I was going. I had goals, and I achieved them."

Joan gave her unwavering dedication to her profession. "To be a successful academic requires a commitment that is greater than in many other jobs. You think about the next steps in your research, or about that student who is struggling, or about that student who is soaring, or about that administrative dilemma in hours that spill over into family time," she explained.

Despite the demanding nature of her work, she really

thrived on solving the daily challenges she faced.   She admittedly never felt thwarted by any problem that was handed to her. She had never been confronted with any "unknown" that threatened to impede her job performance. To the contrary, she approached perplexities with a problem solving mentality and always exhibited confident bearing. She loved her work. Up to this point in her life, she had experienced virtually no extreme challenges that had ever required her to reassess her ideals, her purpose, or the legacy she expected to leave as an academic.

Confronting the Unknown

Then something happened in the year 2000 that changed all of that—she was confronted with the "unknown"—a serious neurological disease that had no known name, and it would turn her world upside down for the next three years. Its progression ultimately forced Joan to resign from her academic profession in 2002.

It was a loss she mourned deeply. Identity, purpose, and legacies were all taken away in one fell swoop. Reflecting on this, she said, "I have always felt [that] it is important to leave a legacy, to somehow leave this world a better place. I have left my career, and up until now, my career has been where I felt that I was leaving my legacy."

However, Joan's resignation was unavoidable. Her condition, ironically, was unaffected by any attempted rehabilitation efforts. "It was a struggle to walk...to organize my thoughts. It was an effort to read, to write, to coordinate my most basic movements. [My body] jerked all the time, [and] I could not control it. My mind was [no longer] as sharp. I [became] slower, and I could no longer remember as well." She could see that her illness had an effect upon her academic associates and others who knew her. "It was hard for them to see me struggling to do things that I once found easy," she said.

She observed in her colleagues' faces, expressions of fear and horrid realization—as if to ask, "What if I was in her position? What would I have in my life without my career?" What a somber thought indeed. Imagine a medical crisis occurring at the pinnacle of one's career and ending everything that had professionally been accomplished through self-sacrifice and hard work. Where is the justice in that?

Joan would not permit herself to dwell long about her loss in those terms. Rather, in characteristic fashion, she sought, first, to problem solve and to identify the mysterious disease that had arrested her body and mind. When did this all begin?

Summer 2000

Her searching thoughts took her back to August of 2000, when she and her husband, Kevin, took a holiday south of Thunder Bay across the border in Michigan and in the Lake of the Woods area. "Kevin and I really enjoyed wilderness canoeing and spent most of our holidays camping and canoeing," Joan said.

She recalled a time, while on this vacation in northern Michigan, when she began to feel ill—a deep, aching pain in her right arm along with overwhelming fatigue and dizziness. When these symptoms did not subside a month later, she made an appointment to consult with her family physician.

At her September appointment, Joan underwent a thorough physical exam, and then her doctor ordered a number of blood tests and x-rays of her chest, neck, shoulder, and humerus. All of the films and test results were unremarkable—everything was negative. Consequently, she was diagnosed with a "sprained right shoulder" and referred to physiotherapy.

However, after a session of physiotherapy, she realized that exercise increased her dizziness and pain, so she returned to her family doctor again and asked to be referred to a neurologist. While she waited for the appointment, her symptoms worsened. "My fatigue was increasing, and the pain in the arm disturbed my sleep. I was losing stamina and could not work a whole day." The appointment with the neurologist could not come soon enough for Joan.

Neurologist

"I truly expected that the neurologist would have the answer on my first visit there. How naive this notion turned out to be," Joan recalled. After an examination, the neurologist said that it appeared as though the pain was referred from another site. Magnetic resonance imaging (MRI) of her full spine was scheduled, and in the interim, Joan was provided with a prescription for pain medication. After the MRI was performed, the images revealed no pathology, only signs of normal aging.

Since her spine was ruled out as a source of Joan's pain, the neurologist ordered an MRI of her brain. These results seriously concerned the doctor and Joan. "This was not normal. There was an area of hyperintensity in the left lateral corpus callosum that suggested possible demyelinating disease." Though this lesion was typical of multiple sclerosis (MS), the criteria for supporting that kind of diagnosis required the presence of more than one lesion.

Although she was not conclusively diagnosed with MS, Joan was still shocked at the presence of a lesion. "I was stunned, but I guess that I believed that this was probably what was wrong with me as my dizziness, fatigue, weakness, and lack of stamina continued." After she returned home again, she began to feel a weakness in the right side of her face accompanied by minor drooling out of the corner of her mouth. To Joan, these latest symptoms seemed to provide additional evidence that she might, indeed, have multiple sclerosis.

Since a diagnosis had so far eluded the neurologist, further tests were ordered. The results were somewhat revealing. "The evoked potential test showed a slowing of responses in the lower limbs, particularly on the left. The first test of the cerebral spinal fluid was negative, meaning no evidence of infections, and oligoclonal bands were normal. My first EEG was also normal," Joan noted. Though relieved that MS was nearly ruled out, Joan and her doctor were still puzzled over the cause of her illness.

Sabbatical

By the fall of 2000, her work responsibilities became nearly impossible for her to perform. She saw the proverbial handwriting on the wall—she had to take time off from work to recuperate. Remembering that she had a sabbatical coming, she decided there was no better time to take it. "I applied for sabbatical, thinking that a year with less to do would be good for my health."

About a week before starting her sabbatical, Joan moved out of the corner office belonging to her as the director of the School of Rehabilitation Sciences and into a professor's office. She rationalized that, though the move was necessary, it did not indicate a permanent loss. After all, she was still the director of the School—the sabbatical did not change that. "It did not feel like the end [of my profession] as I was looking forward to having time to focus on my research. I still could act and think like this was what academics did—they went on sabbatical every few years."

She adapted to the change quickly and philosophically, confident that she would be back at the close of twelve months. Only those colleagues closest to her suspected that something wasn't quite right. They could see she was pale and weak in appearance, and that she was enduring pain. However, most minimized it as stress-induced—something a little time off would surely cure.

Despite their quiet doubts about her health, her peers hosted a grand send off, full of smiles and all the well wishes customary to sabbatical departures. "My colleagues had a surprise dinner at a local restaurant for me. I was truly touched. They gave me a lovely painting, and they all had signed the back with words of appreciation. It did not seem like the end, so there were no tearful goodbyes," she reminisced.

Resignation

Joan returned to her beautiful, suburban home to recuperate and begin her research. She had often thought that her home was a wonderful and welcoming place. Now she had a lot of time to wrap herself in its comfort in hopes that over the next year, she would get well again and return to the work she loved so very much.

However, the sabbatical did not result in a restoration of health as she had initially hoped. In fact, by June 2001, a new and very frightening symptom appeared. "I started to have severe myoclonic jerking (brief, involuntary contractions) in my right hip flexors, which later spread to include my back extensors and then to other muscle groups," she said.

Quickly, she returned to her neurologist, who ordered two MRIs—one of her brain and another of her spine. These images revealed no change from the original ones. Wanting badly to help Joan, her physician prescribed valproic acid, an anticonvulsant that would help control the involuntary jerking. Despite the medication, her sleep was still severely disturbed, and her fatigue worsened even further.

It became clear to Joan that she had some kind of degenerative disease and that she would not be able to return to her office as director. Giving up a job that she so dearly loved caused a deep sadness. Nonetheless, she accepted her reality, and in July 2001, she resigned as the director of the School of Rehabilitation Sciences. "I told my colleagues and my dean that after my sabbatical, I would not be coming back as director. [However], I did not resign as professor at that time," she explained.

A Crossroads

In September, as the new school year was about to commence, Joan came to a further realization. "It became evident as the sabbatical drew to a close that I would not be able to return to work in 2002, so I began sick leave." Up until then, she was able to obscure her illness under the normalcy of a sabbatical; however, her application for sick leave left no doubt as to the reason for her continued absence. "Things could now no longer be seen as normal. I just slipped quietly away as I never really came back from sabbatical—so again, no tearful goodbyes, just a profound feeling of sadness."

As she received the shipment from her office of 37 boxes of personal effects and professional materials, she contemplated the reversal of years of professional achievements. Her losses had become conspicuously measurable, and it aroused in her some soul-searching queries. "I really searched for meaning in my life—to find a new role when all that I worked for was ending," Joan said. A role in life—a place to leave a legacy—was something previously resolved in her mind but now appeared truly gone.

A Neurological Nightmare

It was the fall of 2002, and Joan's illness had still not been diagnosed. Joan recalled, "Every test made it feel like the outcome was going to be terrible. I was devastated by the neuropsychological testing in the fall of 2002." Based on those test results, her neurologist felt that she might be suffering from corticobasal ganglionic degeneration, "a horrible, relentlessly progressive illness where one loses both physical and cognitive abilities before death," explained Joan.

She knew that she could have coped with her physical losses, but this new and morbid diagnosis was almost too much to bear. Joan reacted, "I was tearful most of the time. This was when I truly felt that I was dying and needed to prepare for that. I grieved for the loss of [my] job and for the loss of my future."

Joan's neuromotor dysfunction was becoming more and more pronounced. Walking became unpredictably dangerous since she never knew when the next myoclonic jerk would cause her knees to buckle and collapse beneath her. She explained, "I started to use a cane, first—for safety— then, because I could not walk without it. I [also] began to have difficulties reading. I had nystagmus (involuntary, rhythmic movement of the eyes) and visual pursuit problems." Again, her doctor re-evaluated her medications and changed the anticonvulsant prescription to clonazepam to see if that would offer her some relief. Happily, it did. "The jerking continued but was bearable, and I could now sleep," she said.

In January 2003, Joan's sick leave status ended, and she went on long-term disability. It was another one of those markers in life that documented her continuing decline in health, but it wasn't the only marker Joan remembered. "Cognitive testing revealed acquired brain dysfunction with severe visual memory loss (cortical dysfunction) and some indication of subcortical involvement because of the slowing of information processing, diminished verbal initiation, and memory retrieval."

A second round of tests was performed. First, an EEG showed abnormal, sharp spikes that were unrelated to the myoclonic activity. Then a second spinal tap, which was also abnormal, revealed a mildly positive 14-3-3 protein CSF test. This assay measures the 14-3-3 protein, a marker of central nervous system neuronal injury or death and is used in evaluating Creuztfeldt-Jacob disease. This disease was later ruled out for lack of other defining criteria.

Diagnostic Limbo

Frustrated and puzzled, Joan knew only that she had a progressive neurodegenerative disease, yet her symptoms did not fit the criteria for any known disease of that type. "Differential diagnoses now seemed to be among the so-called Parkinson-Plus syndromes: multiple systems atrophy, progressive supranuclear palsy, or corticobasal ganglionic degeneration," she noted.

Joan acknowledged that from the neurologist's point of view, all known diagnostic tests and evaluations had been thoroughly performed. All known treatable diseases appeared to have been considered. However, the fact remained that her physicians had failed to identify her illness. This state of diagnostic limbo created frustration and allowed further disease progression and delay in any possible treatments.

"It is frustrating and difficult. As a scientist and researcher, I have dealt with concrete data and interpretable results all my life. It is hard to live each day knowing that you have something serious but not knowing how it will progress, how long one might expect to live with this disease, or whether I will need daily help for my every need in two years or twenty," Joan related.

Being without a defined illness left those who knew Joan emotionally perplexed. "It was hard for my family... they were worried, and they did not know how to help. It was hard for them to make their own life decisions not knowing what was happening to me."   Even among her former colleagues, she recalled how they struggled with the concept that she had not yet been diagnosed.

Troubling doubts crept into her mind.   Could her colleagues have been right? Was this illness stress-induced after all?   "I had to reject this notion many times, but the thought kept creeping [back] into my head. [No]—I loved my job. I loved the variety, the unexpected problems, the camaraderie with like-minded individuals, the recognition for my work, and the creative nature of my research. I liked guiding my students in their learning. I did not feel in the least like I was burning out," responded Joan.

The recurrence of self doubt was the most hurtful aspect of being in a diagnostic limbo. She desperately reasoned, "If the experts cannot figure it out, maybe it *is* all in my head!" So Joan sought the advice of a psychologist to try to determine if clinical depression could be the cause of her many symptoms. The psychologist assured Joan that she was someone who had suffered many losses during the past two years and that she was reacting to those losses in a normal way.

Even though clinical depression was ruled out as the cause of her ailments, Joan did feel episodes of profound sadness as might be expected for any normal individual in her situation. She realized that being left without a concrete diagnosis often isolated her from merciful, human understanding. It seemed as though those without a medical background found her predicament beyond comprehension. They were unsure how to act around her, how to comfort her, and so they were not as supportive as they could have been.

Surely, they witnessed her pitiful symptoms, but without that definitive medical label, they could not psychologically produce a feeling of empathy. Why not? Because empathy occurs when a person puts himself in the other person's shoes. This is apparently quite difficult for some to do when they don't know the shoe type or size.

"We all seem to want to put things in boxes, to categorize (e.g. this is a serious problem, or this is not so bad and will get better)," Joan said. She observed that the absence of a diagnosis prohibited individuals from completing this type of mental cataloging. This, in turn, produced immobilizing emotions such as fear, doubt, or even suspicion and did little to elicit support for Joan.

Joan also learned that social support structures were not in place to help those in a diagnostic limbo. After all, support groups are defined according to medical diagnoses, so there seemed to be no place for patients like Joan who had no diagnostic label. "I cannot go to the MS Society or the ALS or the fibromyalgia support group. I do not belong anywhere, so I continue in limbo waiting for some test to confirm the diagnosis or for my physical or mental deterioration to be so obvious as to make a diagnosis easy."

A Proactive Approach

Ultimately, Joan took a more proactive approach to her undiagnosed illness. "I have found support on the Internet by joining virtual support groups based on my symptoms," explained Joan. She also made some of her own professional decisions. "I know as a physical therapist that not doing exercise will only hasten whatever it is that I have, yet exercise increased my symptoms!" Joan said. Since her physical routines only worsened her symptoms of dizziness and myoclonus, she wisely stopped.

As Joan struggled with her new role as a patient of a serious chronic illness, she asked the members of her health care team, friends, and family to be patient and to realize that there were still many gaps in medical knowledge. "There are still many people out there with strange symptoms that do not fit known diagnostic criteria. Help needs to be geared to the person, not to the disease. I know that diagnosis is important for appropriate medical treatment, but it should not be the basis for appropriate social, emotional, physical, spiritual, and community support."

In August 2003, three years after her first symptoms appeared, she was no closer to a diagnosis than she was at the onset. So, in the absence of a diagnosis, Joan decided to give herself one—a Parkinson-Plus disorder. She also began accessing the support of the Parkinson's Society and attending their support group meetings along with some Tai Chi classes. Then she concentrated on improving her fitness levels through physiotherapy based on motor control principles. Although her muscle strength increased from this work, her stamina did not. Constant fatigue, dizziness, and episodes of myoclonus persisted despite physiotherapy.

Psychogenic Source

Finally, in November 2003, Joan decided with great hesitancy, to explore the neurologist's persistent contention that the origin of her illness could be psychogenic. Why a psychogenic disorder? The neurologist explained that this was an illness caused by some deep, psychological process, such as a childhood trauma or some more unthinkable act of victimization.

His professional suggestion seemed repulsive and accusatory. "I know in my heart-of-hearts that this cannot be true, but I feel like a prisoner who has been unjustly accused of a crime." Joan felt compelled to follow through on this matter since it appeared to be a significant impediment to further unbiased treatment by the neurologist.

Consequently, she decided to submit to a psychiatric evaluation in order to determine whether or not there was any truth to the neurologist's claim. When she asked the neurologist to refer her to a psychiatrist—not once but five times—he procrastinated. Upon her first request, the neurologist responded negatively, "A psychiatrist cannot help you." The next time she asked for a referral, the neurologist became even more indignant, "A psychiatrist will talk to you for 45 minutes and determine that you are not depressed and send you back to me saying, 'It is organic.'"

The neurologist's illogic frustrated Joan. On one hand, he insisted she had a psychogenic disorder, but on the other hand, he would not cooperate to have his presumption professionally validated. How could she get him to cooperate? Joan doggedly persevered and eventually was able to secure a referral to consult with a psychiatrist.

The evaluation was completed over the course of two visits, and the resulting psychiatric profile was sent to the neurologist. It read that no psychiatric indications of pathology or clinical depression existed. Needless to say, the neurologist refused to believe that he was wrong.

A Pharmacist's Advice

One day in late November, Joan went to the pharmacy to inquire about supplements that might help her unremitting fatigue. She spoke with the pharmacist about her medical symptoms, and he suggested that she look into Lyme disease. Joan responded, "I had been twice tested for Lyme disease, and the tests were negative." He then suggested that she check out the reliability of the tests she had taken.

When Joan returned home, she did just that. "During the next few days, I checked the literature about testing for Lyme disease, and I was astounded to find out that the screening test can miss up to 70% of those infected with Lyme. I found out that Lyme is a clinical diagnosis and that tests are not to be used to exclude it as a possibility."

After learning this, Joan discovered tests that were more sensitive and reliable for evaluating Lyme disease than the one she had submitted to previously. How grateful she was for the pharmacist's advice.

New Tests for Lyme

In December, Joan met with her general practitioner, a doctor she had known for 15 years. This physician was willing to order Western blot tests for Lyme disease and sent her blood to a U.S. laboratory. The results were positive for Lyme. At this point, Joan's doctor discharged herself from the case because she knew treatment was beyond her level of expertise. She suggested, instead, that Joan consult with an infectious disease (ID) specialist. An appointment was scheduled, although it meant waiting a few months.

While waiting for that appointment, Joan decided to contact the office of a doctor in Vancouver, who routinely treated Lyme disease patients in Canada. Joan wrote to the doctor and sent him her medical history and test results to consider. He accepted her case, and an appointment was made to see him on January 7, 2004.

After a full evaluation by this physician, he advised Joan that, in his opinion, it appeared highly probable that she had Lyme disease. He commenced treatment immediately with two different oral antibiotics. He also stressed that she would have to get the cooperation of her general practitioner in order to schedule appropriate tests to monitor liver function before and during treatment.

This seemed like a simple, straight-forward directive, so she requested the help of her general practitioner. At that consultation on January 9, her doctor refused to do the blood work or to countersign the prescription. Again, she told Joan that chronic Lyme disease required specialized treatment that was beyond her knowledge base.

However, the doctor reminded Joan that since she had an upcoming appointment with an infectious disease doctor, she could ask him to order these tests. Joan had no choice, apparently, so she looked forward to pursuing this matter with the specialist.

A Skeptic

On January 21, Joan met with the infectious disease specialist. Unfortunately, he had only treated one Lyme disease case in the past and demonstrated a strong skepticism about this particular illness. Joan was immediately concerned by his bias and evident lack of experience treating Lyme disease. Joan noted, "He could not interpret the [laboratory] report and said that he wanted to do his own tests."

Joan tried to accept his position, both from a scientific and legal standing, but she also knew the time involved backtracking would mean further delay in treatment. Since she was desperate to find a cooperating physician, she continued to converse with him about her case history.

She recalled, "He said some things about Lyme that were clearly false, but I could not argue with him. For example, when I said that I did not remember a tick bite but was often camping and doing outdoor activities, he told me that I could only be infected by a fully engorged tick that was large—not the poppy seed size or the freckle size that I had seen described in the literature." Serious concerns surfaced in Joan's mind as she listened to him confidently present this misinformation—but that was not all.

When Joan told him that she felt she had been infected in northern Michigan while on a wilderness camping trip, he refuted that assumption. "He told me that I was not camping in an endemic area, as I was not camping at Point Pelee." Joan was aware that studies proved otherwise—that Ontario and the Upper Peninsula area of Michigan, where she first became ill, were endemic for Lyme disease.

She quietly listened to his presentation of Lyme disease "facts," and afterward, he proceeded to schedule some diagnostic tests. First, the doctor ordered a blood draw and tests for Lyme disease. Then, he asked her to return for a follow-up consultation in six weeks. With that accomplished, Joan left his clinic but not without serious doubts about this physician's ability to perform in a role beneficial to her as a Lyme disease patient.

The next day, Joan consulted with another family practitioner since her own family doctor felt unqualified to treat her. This new physician, a man who had a local practice, listened to Joan talk about her medical history and her present concerns about the ID specialist.

He suggested that Joan go to an experienced U.S. Lyme disease doctor, whom he knew from attending several conferences. The general practitioner knew that this specialist had a large Lyme practice in New York, and Joan would find help there. He arranged an appointment for Joan with this physician for the following day, January 23.

Without further delay, Joan and Kevin drove through the night until they arrived 11 hours later at the clinic in the U.S. "I was seen by [the doctor] for an hour and a half, and I was at his clinic for more than four hours," recalled Joan. She provided a thorough record of her case history after which the specialist conducted a physical examination. She also had blood samples drawn that were immediately sent to several U.S. laboratories which specialized in Lyme disease testing to substantiate the original positive test results.

Based upon his clinical examination and review of her case history, which included positive lab results for Lyme disease, the physician was confident that Joan had active Lyme infection. Finally, Joan appeared to have a firm label for her illness, and a treatment protocol was discussed. "The [doctor] said that I should be treated aggressively for Lyme disease and said that he would inform [my general practitioner] that I should receive at least eight weeks of intravenous (IV) Rocephin." The doctor also planned on introducing another antibiotic, Zithromax, one week after IV therapy started.

Physicians Three

Joan felt fortunate to have networked a team of three cooperating physicians with whom she could consult and receive treatment. The Lyme disease specialist who made the diagnosis and was willing to provide guidance was going to play a key role in her treatment. The general practitioner and the infectious disease doctor, who lived in closer proximity to her, would administer the treatment and monitor her health throughout.

The first part of her treatment protocol involved the insertion of a PICC line (peripherally inserted central catheter) so that IV Rocephin could be administered to Joan. A PICC line must be inserted into a peripheral vein, usually in the arm, and carefully advanced so that the tip remains in the large vein just above the heart (superior vena cava). This device can remain in place for a long period of time and is used for administering an extended course of IV medicine.

"[My general practitioner] felt that it would be best if the infectious disease specialist ordered the PICC line and supervised the first treatment. The Community Care Access Centre (CCAC) would then come into my home daily to administer the treatment," explained Joan.

Joan's appointment with the ID doctor was set for February 17, but when she asked the clinic's secretary if the PICC line would be installed at that time, the secretary didn't know. "The secretary said she would ask the doctor and get back to me. [However] she did not call back.   I phoned the [doctor's] secretary [again] and asked about the PICC line. She said that the doctor was waiting for his test results and only wanted to see me. There would be no PICC line [installed] on that date."

Disappointed, Joan began to wonder whether or not this doctor was going to cooperate in treating her. She sensed a last minute hesitancy on his part and wondered why he would delay treatment when the U.S. Lyme disease specialist had made a firm diagnosis that included supportive laboratory evidence. Earlier, he seemed willing to cooperate, but now, Joan had her doubts about him.

Five days before her appointment with the ID specialist, she received a call from the clinic in New York. The Lyme disease specialist informed Joan that the results from the additional tests he had ordered had come back positive for Lyme. Then he asked her how her IV therapy was progressing. She told him that it had not started because the ID specialist had not installed the PICC line.

Puzzled, he volunteered to call the reluctant physician and inquire about this delay in treatment. The two professionals conferred together, and ultimately the ID doctor agreed to install the PICC line as a "professional courtesy" to his colleague. Joan's general practitioner called the ID doctor, and he felt certain that the PICC line would be installed at her next appointment on the 17th of February. At last, everything seemed to be in place for the initial phase of her treatment.

Confronting Opposition

With some remaining reservations about the February visit, Joan decided to bring along her husband, Kevin, as her advocate. The experience turned out to be not only uncomfortable but decidedly strange. "My husband and I waited 45 minutes in an empty waiting room, then [we] were ushered into an exam room. [The doctor] came in with his nurse to act as a witness," Joan recalled.

The news was not good. The doctor informed Joan that he would not treat her for Lyme disease because the results from the Canadian lab came back negative. She recalled his shocking words, "Based on these results and the fact that you were not camping in an endemic area, making the probability of Lyme disease low, I cannot be involved in any way in your treatment."

Kevin asked him how he could ignore the positive PCR (polymerase chain reaction) and Western blot test results from the U.S. laboratories along with the medical opinions of two Lyme disease specialists. The doctor alluded to liability issues when he told them that he could not treat Joan without his own diagnosis. He also warned against the risks involved in treating without adequate medical evidence. Kevin countered that argument by reminding him that a Lyme disease diagnosis is made clinically and includes supportive laboratory results—all criteria that were met in Joan's case. The practitioner's reply to this logic seemed unintelligible to both Joan and Kevin.

Noticing their frustration, the ID specialist suggested that Joan repeat some of the same tests performed by the U.S. labs. She could see no logic or reason to this suggestion other than further delaying treatment, so she refused. To appease her and direct attention away from himself as the deserting physician, he told her that her general practitioner had agreed to install the PICC line and to supervise the first treatment.

Joan was surprised to hear this since her doctor had always deferred to a specialist for the treatment of Lyme disease. In any case, Joan realized that as of that moment, her doctor-patient relationship was terminated with this physician. She would have to continue searching for someone who would be willing to treat her.

A Patient's Quandary

Momentarily, Joan reassessed what had transpired so far in her case history. "I am positive by CDC criteria on the IgG and IgM done [in the U.S.]. I have a positive PCR for Lyme from [another U.S.] lab. I have seen two doctors specializing in Lyme, and both say that I have Lyme disease. [Despite this,] I cannot get treatment! It does not seem that the Canadian lab has the expertise to do testing for Lyme disease, and Canadian doctors are not respecting the American lab results. How can the Canadian lab results come back negative when I am clearly positive with respected U.S. labs?" she wondered.

Joan wanted a copy of those Canadian lab reports. She called her general practitioner's office and was told that the doctor did not have the detailed reports yet, but that as soon as she had them, she would send a copy to Joan. She also inquired about when the physician would install a PICC line to begin her treatment. There was a pause, and then the secretary said that the doctor would have to call her later to discuss that matter with her.

Now that the ID specialist had withdrawn his participation in her treatment, Joan feared that her doctor would also refuse to treat her. After all, if an infectious disease doctor refused to treat her for lack of positive test results from Canadian labs, why would a general practitioner comply?

"I was in trouble because I could not get any other doctor to go against the advice of the ID [specialist] and order a PICC...and the doctors in the hospital would not go against their colleague." Joan knew that if she was going to continue to receive her physician's help, the U.S. Lyme disease specialist would have to become more supportive.

Finally, Joan received the long-awaited, return phone call from her general practitioner. During their conversation, the doctor denied that she had told the ID specialist that she would install the PICC and supervise the first treatment. She explained that it was impossible for her to do that procedure because she did not have the necessary hospital privileges. Beyond disappointment and amazed at the creativity of this endless run-around, Joan immediately called the U.S. Lyme disease specialist for help.

All the while, the medical bills and expenses were mounting, and she had not even begun treatment. Laboratory bills, doctor visit bills, travel and phone expenses—these were all costs that Joan or her national healthcare insurance would have to pay.

Canadian Healthcare

The Canadian National Healthcare system is a single tier system. There are no private insurance companies that pay for hospital or doctor visits or other essential services in Canada. Joan had insurance that covered mostly prescription drugs, but other than that, she relied upon the national healthcare system like any other Canadian citizen.

In her quest for treatment, Joan had incurred over $10,000 in medical expenses which the Canadian healthcare system refused to pay. "I had to pay out-of-pocket for Lyme disease testing in the U.S. I [also] had to pay for my visits to the Lyme disease doctor in New York and my telephone consultations with him. I was not covered for any of the supplements that I took, which added up to about $250 a month or for the extra testing that my family doctor [ordered] to check my neurotransmitter levels," Joan explained.

Admittedly, these out-of-pocket expenses represented a small fraction of the total cost involved in treating her case of disseminated Lyme disease. "All of my doctors' visits here in Canada were covered as were the daily nursing visits while I was on the IV [therapy]. The cost of the Rocephin was also covered by the healthcare system as I was under home care which is covered by the system."

The cost of the installation of the PICC at the U.S. hospital (over $2,000) was not covered by the Canadian healthcare system; however, "there was no problem getting the nine weeks of IV [therapy] once I had the PICC and my general practitioner ordered the treatment. It was never questioned."

Treatment Begins

Initially, Joan seemed to be at an impasse when it came to finding a physician who would install the necessary PICC line. Eventually, with a great deal of persistence and perseverance, Joan was able to gain her general practitioner's cooperation in implementing an alternative plan. He agreed to supervise the administration of her first dose of IV Rocephin at his office on February 26, 2004, using a peripheral venous line instead of a PICC. The distinct disadvantage to this route was that every three days, the line had to be removed and a new sterile line had to be reinserted into a new vein. The discomforts involved with this mode of administration were weighed by Joan, and she felt that the peripheral line was better than forestalling the treatment altogether, so she willingly submitted to this route.

Further daily treatments were arranged through the

home care agency and administered by nurses at Joan's home. At first, her daily treatments at home seemed to proceed without any problems. However, it wasn't long before the nurses began to experience difficulty finding available veins for the peripheral line. Finally, this route of administration became impossible. "The PICC almost became an emergency [issue] as it was either stop treatment or get a PICC," Joan explained.

Hesitantly, she called the ID specialist and asked him, once again, if he would install a PICC so that she could continue her treatment. She assured him that the general practitioner was taking full responsibility for the treatment and that she was only requesting his cooperation with regard to the installing of the PICC. Nothing she said made any difference—he flatly refused to help her.

Wasting no time, Joan contacted the Lyme practitioner in New York and made firm arrangements for a PICC to be installed at his office. Joan and Kevin immediately drove there for this procedure so that treatment could continue. "Unfortunately, the nurse could not insert it after trying for over an hour. [The doctor] sent me to the local hospital, and the PICC was put in by a radiologist." Sore and mentally and physically exhausted, Joan traveled home the following day.

Improvements Noted

Joan immediately resumed IV therapy and finished it on April 27. Following this therapy, she continued on oral antibiotics. In addition to using antibiotics, she also employed a few complementary approaches to boost her immune system and restore any nutrient depletion. She began to routinely take a daily multivitamin along with vitamin B-12 injections twice weekly. The combination, she thought, would help strengthen her body so that it could overcome the infection more readily and heal her nervous system.

One month later, she noted a remarkable improvement in her health. "I was starting to get better. I could read again! My balance was better. The jerking had nearly stopped. My walking had improved, and I no longer needed my cane to walk!"

It was a notable upturn in Joan's condition. For four years prior to treatment, she had been plagued by disabling symptoms. "I could only walk a few feet with the help of a cane. I was constantly jerking. I had cognitive problems (spatial and facial recognition problems, loud noise intolerance, and concentration difficulties). I was so weak. I could not lift my leg off the bed or lift more than one pound weights with my arms. I could not coordinate my movements, and I had severe balance difficulties with very little hope of ever getting better."

After five months of treatment, Joan was beginning to enjoy life again. "I am over the moon about my progress. I can walk around the block without my cane. I am stronger and more coordinated. I can stand on one foot without falling over. I am still getting stronger every day, and there is still the worry that I may relapse when I finish the antibiotics, but for the moment, I am savoring better health. It is sweet!"

In July 2004, Joan was taken off all of her antibiotics. "I am holding my own. I still take supplements. Physically, I am really very good. There are still some remaining cognitive issues which may prevent my return to work as university professor. I am hoping these continue to resolve."

Long Term Disability

On November 18, Joan met with a psychologist for neuropsychological retesting. The last time Joan had gone through this type of testing was two years earlier, so she hoped that this time there would be some evidence of improvement.

But after six hours of testing, Joan suspected that she had not progressed much since her last test. "The kinds of things I found difficult two years ago, I still found difficult," she said. Anticipating that the doctor would share the results with her then, she inquired. To her surprise, he told her that he could not share the information with her yet.

He explained that before she would be allowed to learn the results of his evaluation, his report had to be sent to the insurance company. Joan was shocked that the patient, in essence, was not entitled to be the first informed. With no other choice, she waited for further news about her test results.

Three weeks later, the insurance company called and said that, based upon the neuropsychological evaluation, they officially judged Joan as "disabled" and would continue to pay her long-term disability. This report was faxed to Joan's doctor and forwarded to her on December 17, 2004. She read it slowly and thought about its many somber implications.

For someone who wanted to return to work, this wasn't what Joan wanted to read. She responded, "It made me very sad that I could have so much improvement physically while hardly improving at all cognitively." The cognitive difficulties she referred to included multitasking, word finding, fatigability, visual memory, and reading challenges.

Despite these major disabilities, she was not going to give up. "I am left to try to figure out the next steps. Do I try to find a purpose without my work at the university? Do I try to have more treatment?" Joan's mind was bombarded with questions. "I guess what I do not know is if this is still Lyme or is it damage from Lyme. I feel so good in all other respects. I just do not know what to think."

Joan had much to contemplate. She planned to consult with her Lyme doctor about her questions and about further treatment options. She also intended to explore alternative treatments. She said, "I am not despairing as I now have a much better quality of life than a year ago. It may be that after all that has happened to me, that academia is not the place I want to be anymore. I do need to find something that is rewarding to do...but I will figure it out."

A Professor's Lessons

It could be said that serious illness is the most uncompromising of life's schoolmasters. Its lessons are forcefully taught; its students indiscriminately selected. Its legacies are boldly and indelibly etched into mind, heart, and flesh. That was the experience of Professor Joan McComas, after she was forced to leave the world of academics to become a student of a different sort.

Noting the most difficult of her lessons, she said, "I have learned not to trust doctors so much. This was a hard lesson for me as I was part of that system. I learned that you have to take charge of your own health [in order] to get better." Joan felt that the implicit trust she once placed in the medical establishment was a misplaced trust.

Joan learned that physicians may have limited or no working knowledge of certain diseases. She found that obstacles can be placed in a patient's way to make access to help even more difficult because a doctor wants to avoid dealing with specific disorders. The patient ends up floundering in the muddle and must somehow bear the burden of physician inability and bias—usually unacknowledged—and the disease simultaneously. Only dogged persistence, self education, and refusal to give up or give in keep one from falling through the cracks in medicine.

In addition, Joan observed serious weaknesses in the healthcare system itself—not to mention the plight of the international patient—and add to that the burden of finding competent medical care. In Canada, as in other countries, those with little money are truly left to whatever their particular system wishes to offer. It is a sobering reality.

On a very personal level, Joan learned what cannot be taught in an academic forum or research laboratory. She learned how it personally felt to have one's physical health and vitality taken away—that along with one's professional identity. Joan, who was once a highly respected professor and researcher at the university, had enjoyed a privileged life as a successful academic. It was a good life, a secure life, and she knew exactly who she was and where she would leave her legacies.

Just as quickly, though, everything she had worked for was dismantled, boxed up, and sent home to her for storage. Her physical prowess was reduced to that of a homebound patient with severe disabilities. What happened? Told only that she had a progressive neurological disorder and that it was incurable was devastating. When nearly all hope was robbed from her, and a diagnosis still eluded the doctors consulted, she was made the scapegoat—"You have a psychogenic disorder."

Joan felt it was professional cruelty at its worst. However, as soon as the diagnosis was made and treatment begun, good health gradually returned to Joan, and along with it, a sense of personal and professional vindication. This reversal of circumstances, though, meant yet another adjustment emotionally. She said of her near-death to life transformation, "The adjustment for a person who is dying from an unknown neurological illness to one who is getting better is huge. I am making that adjustment now. Who knows how far I will go, but I have come a long, long way. I am a different person now."

She truly is a different person, one whose figurative eyes see life, health, and love in a philosophically expansive way. "I have learned to adapt and to cope with things that I never thought I would have to cope with. I have learned that I can be resilient. I have learned to reflect more about the bigger questions in life, [and] I have slowed down."

Joan applied herself to the study of her symptoms, and once diagnosed, she became a student of Lyme disease, its politics, history, and science. She assertively took charge of her own health, and it paid off. "It has been a test of determination," she explained.

After four years of suffering with Lyme disease, Joan cautions others who are experiencing similar symptoms to "consider Lyme disease as a possibility." She advises others to go to different doctors and to be your own advocate. "Find out about testing and get tested at a lab specializing in Lyme disease."

With regard to dealing with medical healthcare providers, she said, "Develop a tough skin because you will be told, 'no', and 'it's all in your head', and 'there is nothing I can do for you.' If you do not feel right about what you are being told, keep seeking. Do not give up. Diagnosis is just the first step."

Treatment may be psychologically welcoming, but Joan was candid about this too. "Treatment [can be] long and hard, and there will be days that you will feel like you are not getting anywhere. Develop a support system, online and in real life. It helps!" This is exactly what she had done, and her family rallied around her.

Joan's Legacies

Five years earlier, when she first became ill, she may have wondered, *What would I have in my life without my career?* She thought performing well in her career would be her most prominent legacy in life. Without doubt, she did leave a legacy with the university's science and rehabilitation departments, but that wasn't the most prominent one.

In the darkest days of her illness, Joan discovered her true legacy in life. It was right in front of her all the time, disguised perhaps, but it was there. In fact, a colleague brought it to her attention with the questioning prose of "Late Fragment" by Raymond Carver.

And did you get what
you wanted from this life, even so?
I did.
And what did you want?
To call myself beloved, to feel myself
beloved on the earth.

Joan McComas learned that to experience love was really her greatest legacy in life. "I have had a charmed life, and I can call myself beloved and do feel beloved on this earth." She wondered if she felt beloved because of her accomplishments, her relationships, or just because of being who she was. She knows now that she is beloved for all of those things because they are all expressions of her heart.

"I have left a legacy at the university and in my profession. I am proud of what I have accomplished. I [also] think my children are part of my legacy. It is good to see them functioning well, well-educated, in good jobs, and in happy relationships. Part of my legacy has been to help them to adulthood," she reflected.

As for the future, Joan can only wonder. "I am now struggling with the 'what now?' questions. I am not sure what my post-Lyme legacy will be. I know that I help people with Lyme, who contact me, and I will become more involved in the Canadian Lyme Foundation. I still cannot see past these things."

Whatever happens beyond this, Joan McComas,

Ph.D., is resolved to turn her circumstances into a loving expression of herself. After all, it is mankind's greatest gift. She explained, "I loved and was loved in return. That is what I treasure most—'To call myself beloved, to feel myself beloved on earth.'"

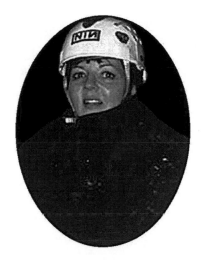

Sue

Contest for Mind and Soul

"Out of suffering have emerged
the strongest souls."
—*Edwin Hubbell Chapin*

At eight years of age, Sue Ferguson of Vancouver Island, British Columbia, made her debut as a competing athlete in the equine arena. Five years later, she was participating in almost every division of the Equine Canadian Nationals. By the time she was 16, she was a qualified riding instructor who taught, trained, judged, and traveled to give clinics. "When I wasn't traveling the show circuit, I was out trail riding or climbing mountains or involved in some kind of outdoor activity," said Sue.

As an adult, she became predominantly occupied with climbing. "In later years, I became obsessed with rock and ice climbing and spent every available moment hiking up steep trails all over the country in search of good climbing areas," Sue said. Every available moment meant those times when she wasn't working full time adjudicating insurance claims for her employer or when she wasn't actively engaged in her duties as wife and mother in her family life.

It was certainly a balancing act of sorts, but she never felt more mentally or physically fit to handle it. "[I] led a very full and happy social life. Energy was never an issue. I was passionate about my job and my life outside of work. Everything flowed," she reminisced.

Island Environment

Living on the southern tip of Vancouver Island, Sue was aware of the fact that Lyme disease had been reported to occur in the area. She recalled, "I had once picked up [a brochure on Lyme disease] out of curiosity from a travel clinic that talked about LymeRix (a Lyme vaccine that is no longer sold), and it listed two places in Canada as being Lyme endemic: Vancouver Island, [including] the west coast of the mainland, and Point Pele in Ontario."

In her area of the island, she was constantly pulling ticks off her clothing, yet she admits, "When I think back on it, [I] never associated them with becoming very ill. Encountering lots of ticks was just part of being out in the bush." In fact, there were times during the year when their prolific numbers were alarming. This was particularly evident in the early spring when they would seem to "rain" from the trees.

It was a common occurrence for Sue to flick them off her clothes or backpack while she was mountain biking or rock climbing. As an added precaution, she followed a routine to rid herself of them when she came in from outdoors. "It was routine practice to come home from climbing and immediately throw everything into the dryer to kill any ticks that might be on my clothing."

Despite these precautionary habits, the odds were that one day she would come face-to-face with a serious tick bite incident. That day came in March 2000 after a full day of rock climbing on a local mountain. "We were climbing four or five days a week, so [the tick] might have been there a day or two, but I assumed it had only been there since early that morning. I was taking my hair out of a ponytail, [when] I felt a lump just behind my ear at the hairline. It felt odd, so I checked it out in the mirror. It was a fully engorged tick!" Sue explained.

Being instantly repulsed by it, she squeezed it between her fingers and yanked it off her skin. Several hours later, Sue's immune system went into a heightened response. "That night I woke up in the middle of the night, drenched in sweat, feverish, and [I] started [to] vomit," She explained. Sue thought this was very unusual for her since the last time she had the flu was more than ten years before. Later, she realized that by squeezing the tick's engorged body, as she had done, it disgorged its content straight into her system.

Initial Doctor's Visit

The next day, she went in to see her doctor, bringing the tick with her. The doctor decided to forward it along with a sample of Sue's blood to the lab for preliminary Lyme disease testing. Meanwhile, he prescribed an antibiotic for her to take until the lab reports came back and a diagnosis could be made. "My doctor put me on doxycycline and sent me home," she said. Doxycycline is an antibiotic frequently used as a first defense against Lyme and several other tick-borne diseases. However, side effects can occur if one is sensitive to the tetracycline family of drugs. In Sue's case, she quickly developed a stomach ache after her first few doses, so she quit taking the medicine.

Unaccustomed to being sick, Sue grew impatient with the treatment and said, "I felt the doxycycline made me feel worse than the tick bite did; and besides, I was too busy to be sick. I got over it and didn't give it another thought. I threw the pills into a drawer and forgot about them." Sue felt certain that whatever made her ill had passed and would not recur.

When the blood test results came back from the lab, they were negative for Lyme disease. The lab also noted that since the tick had been squeezed by the patient, there was an insufficient sample size to perform testing. So with that outcome and seemingly improved health, Sue put the matter behind her and was sent home without further instructions.

No one seemed to realize, however, that Lyme disease testing cannot reveal anything this early in the disease process; in other words, ordering a Lyme test a few days after the bite was an error that can lead to a false negative result. The antibodies to the Lyme spirochete that are measured by these tests take weeks to develop. This key point was entirely overlooked or, perhaps, never understood to begin with by the physician in charge. While a patient would not be expected to know this, a medical professional who employs such tests should.

Bull's-Eye

About one week later, Sue noticed a large, red, ring-shaped rash near the area where the tick had bitten her. "It extended down onto my neck," Sue explained. She wondered what was causing this rash and thought it was odd that the rash would appear so late after the tick bite occurred. She did not know that the initial erythema migrans (EM) rash of Lyme disease can show up weeks—appearing most often 3 to 30 days—following the bite. Maybe it was there earlier.

Perhaps she just hadn't seen it behind her ear and under her hair until now. Whatever the case, Sue ignored it, and it disappeared within a few weeks.

Admittedly, at the time, she never thought about researching Lyme disease to see if her rash had any medical significance, and her physician never alerted her to report any signs or symptoms that might develop with time. She thought about it later. "In hindsight, Lyme disease was glaring," she said. The signs were there, but she never gave it any thought once the rash disappeared. The initial Lyme rash can be used—without test confirmation—to diagnose a case of Lyme disease. Had she been advised by a knowledgeable practitioner, she would have promptly reported this rash to a physician and sought immediate treatment. Unfortunately for Sue, these simple, avoidable medical errors later led to major problems for her.

Over the following two years, Sue started to develop unexplainable aches and pains resembling arthritis. She reasoned, "I just assumed the arthritis was from old sports injuries, or that I was pushing myself too hard physically."

In 2001, Sue had taken her sports to a new level. She was training rigorously with a team for adventure racing. She put in over 30 hours a week in training for all the different disciplines. She explained how she managed to do this with the arthritic pain she was enduring. "I was able to push through bone and joint pain with anti-inflammatories. I had always been ultra healthy, so I think my immune system just kept everything under control during this time."

Severe Flu

By the time the racing season ended in August of 2001, Sue was tired and worn out. She no longer had the motivation to pursue many of her athletic interests. "I remember not wanting to do anything (climbing, kayaking, hiking). [It was] too demanding, and [I] just was doing lots of casual mountain biking and road riding for fun."

Then in October, Sue experienced a serious injury when she was biking down a steep rock face. "My tire skidded out on the wet moss, and rather than go down, I slipped out and went over the cliff to the right. I was airborne for about 15 feet, hit my head on a stump, fractured my wrist and hurt my back," she explained.

Within less than a month after this trauma to her body, she came down with what appeared to be a severe flu. "I couldn't move my neck [because] my headache was so bad. I couldn't be examined. It was the first time I remember feeling as though my brain was being squeezed out of my ears!" Sue said. She experienced severe backache and pain in her ankles, knees, feet, wrists, and jaw.

By November, Sue's doctor suspected that she had Lyme disease. Her blood was drawn and sent to a lab for testing, using a simple antibody test called ELISA. The Canadian CDC was informed, but the results came back negative. Consequently, for the second time, Lyme disease was ruled out, and it wasn't given a second thought by Sue or her physician. It did not seem to occur to the doctor that test results are only a part of the clinical work-up—that they should not be what a diagnosis relies on exclusively—and that the ELISA is not without controversy as to its reliability.

Leave of Absence

Following this "super flu," however, Sue began to experience constant symptoms of severe fatigue and malaise. "My performance at work started to plummet. I just felt really rotten, but I thought I was just exhausted from a year of constantly pushing myself to the physical limit," Sue said.

In December, Sue's condition had notably declined. "I was so run down, my mother said I looked like the walking dead." Every morning Sue woke with red, sore, and goopy eyes. She also experienced severe joint, neck, and back pain. Looking for some kind of physical relief, she tried massage and physiotherapy, but nothing seemed to help.

With failure confronting her at every turn, Sue's emotions started to buckle beneath the stress. "I started to have a lot of anxiety issues about being so tired all of the time and not being able to keep up at work and being worn down by being in constant pain." With few choices remaining, Sue put in for a leave of absence from work. It was hard for her to believe that she once led her co-workers in lunch hour aerobics work-outs, and now she was unable to move a single joint without great pain.

During her leave of absence, she had two other accidents, the latter of which required reconstructive ligament surgery. After these accidents, Sue had to go on sick leave from work. "That caused a lot of problems with my employer. It was an extremely stressful time," Sue remembered.

Ever hopeful, Sue set a personal goal to get well in time to train for and participate in two different athletic events the following year: mountain biking and road riding. Her surgeon assured her that she would be well enough to train and race the following season and would even be back to ice climbing the following winter. After all, she was admitted for surgery as "an athlete with a bad leg injury." No one knew any differently.

Cognitive Impairment

When Sue woke up from that surgery, things were

never the same again. She experienced unremitting fatigue. "I can't describe the depth of the exhaustion. At first, it was like I had been injected with anesthesia. I could hardly hold my head up. Nothing made sense anymore. I just didn't seem to grasp the meaning of what people were saying to me. I was extremely emotional, crying all of the time."

Suddenly, Sue was in the athletic event of her life, and the starting flags had already been waved. There was no turning back, no stopping the clock, and it was going to be an uphill race for life itself. If her post-operative recovery was any indicator, she had started her race for life with a big handicap—profound fatigue and mental confusion.

Trying to explain this phenomenon, her surgeon suggested that perhaps she had experienced an allergic reaction to the anesthesia, and if so, it would lift within three months. However, it did not lift at all. Meanwhile, she rested at home, and when friends came to visit her, she could tolerate only a brief visit. "Within minutes, I became so exhausted that I would have to tell them to leave [so] I [could] go to bed."

In addition to fatigue, Sue felt an odd head sensation. "The exhaustion was accompanied [by] the strangest kind of head pressure. It [was] like an egg yolk sticking to the back of the shell, and that is how my brain was. It felt solid and unwilling to give me anything to work with, to be able to have a meaningful conversation with people," Sue tried to explain.

With such intense headaches and head pressure, cognitive functions involving any level of concentration, analyzing, or comprehension would result in dizziness and such exhaustion that she had to stop whatever she was doing and retire to her bed for rest. During this debilitating period, going to the physiotherapist was all Sue could do in a day. Then she returned home to her bed.

An Athlete's Resolve

In spite of her condition, the athlete in her kept pushing to exercise. She tried cycling and swimming, but she noticed serious dysfunction in her motor skills. "My brain was just not connecting to my [injured] leg, and I was not healing nearly as quickly as expected. I was having problems walking and standing. I felt as though I had no strength in either of my legs, and they [felt] exhausted."

Still, the hope of participating in the two racing events the following year spurred her on. "I felt I had to keep going [to] be healthy enough to start training when the time came," Sue said. Wasting no time, she hired a personal trainer and met him regularly at the local gym. He observed her cognitive difficulties at each training session. "He used to say that I appeared to be clawing my way through a fog just trying to make sense of things."

The gym where she met for training was a place where she had previously spent hundreds of hours working out, yet none of it looked familiar to her now. "I no longer knew how to use [the] machines at the gym. I was just out of it," Sue said. The constant mental haze that she experienced caused heightened anxiety, and the anxiety seemed to result in even more confusion. She felt trapped in a vicious cycle, and her self-confidence was greatly diminished.

Back to Work

After four months had passed, Sue felt that she just had to return to her job. However, she was not at all confident that she could handle the responsibilities. She still had difficulty walking. "I could not get extension in my left leg, and [I] had problems with flexion contractures, which were excruciatingly painful," Sue said. In addition to her physical limitations, she still had severe psychoneurological challenges. "Everything seemed to be incredibly busy and noisy. I couldn't bear the noise of the office. I was so hypersensitive to noise, at times, [that] I would just sit and hold my head. It felt like spears being driven into my brain."

Also, Sue found it difficult to remember what it was that she was supposed to do at her job. She could not perform mathematical computations, which were a critical part of her duties in the claims department. Any kind of complex thinking process sent her immediately into what she described as "head implosions." This was always followed by profound fatigue and required bed rest.

Even more troubling to her was the fact that she did not recognize some of her co-workers. Once, she asked questions about an event that happened years ago, thinking it happened during the months she was absent. "I asked [co-workers] about their maternity leave, only to be reminded their children were now in school. I was absolutely out of it," Sue recalled. Simple conversations were shrouded with noise. "I could not understand what they were saying. I [heard] noise and watched their mouths moving, but [I] did not understand the content."

Before she returned to work, Sue went to rehabilitation therapy for her leg and back problems, but once she returned to work, she no longer had time for that. By the end of the work day, she felt awful. "Many days I would come home and just crawl up my stairs and fall into bed in my work clothes. [I was] not even able to get it together enough to call for take out. I could no longer remember how to make meals or even make protein shakes [to] take care of myself," Sue said. Confused and anxious, she had no idea why her brain would not function. She just knew something was seriously wrong.

Seeking Professional Help

In March 2003, while leaving work, she ran into one of the doctors with whom she worked. She proceeded to tell him about her symptoms, and he suggested that she might have "post surgical chronic fatigue syndrome." Sue knew nothing about chronic fatigue syndrome (CFS)—or as it is also called—chronic fatigue and immune dysfunction syndrome (CFIDS). As an athlete, she was familiar with orthopedic injuries and trauma, but she admittedly knew little about diseases or internal medicine. It was obviously time to seek someone knowledgeable in those areas of healthcare.

That same month of March, Sue quit her job and went home to recuperate. "By this time, I was so cumulatively fatigued that I slept for about three weeks. During my waking hours, I was plagued with severe headaches, and I was losing my vision in my right eye." This was just the beginning of an onslaught of frightening symptoms. She said, "I had itching, crawling skin sensations, and rashes. I could not cope with any kind of stress whether it be positive or negative. Everything had to be kept very quiet as I was so hypersensitive to noise [that] even the sound of an opening door hurt my head. I became allergic to fumes, perfumes, and anything chemical."

The orthopedic surgeon who had previously operated on her leg advised Sue that he was certain, after this length of time, her problems were not related to the anesthesia. However, that was as far as his certainty went. He had no idea what was causing her motor dysfunction or other bizarre, neurological symptoms.

She then consulted with a naturopath who tested her for various allergies and discovered that she was allergic to oak. Consequently, she had all of the trees growing close to her house cut away regardless of the species. She also bought air purifiers for the rooms in her home and a double hepa filter vacuum cleaner to reduce dust allergens. She had the carpets torn out in her home and put allergy covers on her mattress and pillows.

Lastly, because she could not tolerate anything scented, she switched all her soaps and detergents to the hypoallergenic types and stopped wearing make-up. Despite all these changes, her health did not improve.

At the next appointment with the naturopath, she was placed on a regimen of nutritional supplements to build up her adrenal system, but they made her ill instead. The naturopath then suggested a cleansing diet, but that also made Sue incredibly sick, so she stopped doing that, too. It seemed oddly contrary to logic that her ill body was violently rejecting any healthful nutrients.

Sue then consulted with a chiropractor whom she had seen in the past. "[The chiropractor] felt that my nervous system was all out of whack and that I would get better if we could balance everything. He also suspected cumulative head trauma, and he [did] a lot of cranial work. That helped with the headaches," Sue recalled.

Meanwhile, Sue had been continuing a weekly routine of massage and physiotherapy for her leg and joint pain. "I tried many types of alternative massage type therapies which did not help. What seemed to help me the most was having my head "squeezed" by the massage therapist or the chiropractor. My headaches would lessen for a while but would just return again."

Finally, Sue sought out a psychologist who specialized in cases of chronic fatigue syndrome. Together they discussed the possible benefits of biofeedback treatments. Just as she was about to try this kind of therapy, Sue's general practitioner contacted her to suggest that she see a neurologist that he highly recommended. Sue agreed, and she never returned to the psychologist.

Sue's search for professional help had thus far led her to several specialists, none of whom had been able to diagnose her illness. She tried natural therapies and pharmaceutical treatments, yet she only had increasing symptoms and more pain. All of this was costly, and with depleted savings, she was now managing her healthcare on borrowed funds. Despite this, she could not afford to give up. From this climber's perspective, she was between a rock and a hard place, and there was no way out but up.

Chronic Fatigue Syndrome

Two months had passed since she had left her job, and it was May 2003. Sue's appointment with the neurologist finally arrived, and all kinds of anticipatory thoughts raced through her mind. Sue said, "I was wondering if maybe I had been hit on the head too many times from falling off of horses and bikes or something. I expected her to say that I had post concussion syndrome."

Instead, much to Sue's horror, the neurologist told her that she exhibited signs of multiple sclerosis. Sue responded, "It had never occurred to me that I would have something like this." The doctor ordered some nerve tests and a brain MRI. The results of the brain MRI showed some lesions but no evidence of demyelination. In response to the test results, the neurologist modified her first diagnosis and told Sue that she had chronic fatigue syndrome with primary cognitive dysfunction. The doctor prescribed Provigil for fatigue, and Sue was sent home.

Provigil is a central nervous system stimulant used to help fight fatigue and increase locomotor activity among other therapeutic effects. However, for Sue, Provigil had serious side effects that she was unable to tolerate. "This drug threw me into extreme anxiety and agitation, and I had really bad rashes," she said. The doctor then prescribed Elavil, but it caused problems, too. Discouraged, Sue said, "I seemed to be intolerant to any kind of drug or supplement."

Her health had deteriorated into a deplorable state. Brain functions, including memory recall, were greatly diminished. She experienced more frequent episodes of disorientation and confusion, and severe fatigue was a daily affliction. In addition to these symptoms, other disturbing conditions appeared from March to July. First, she noticed that she was losing her ability to speak properly. Her face was going numb on the left side, and she was constantly drooling. Then, the vision through her right eye became blurry, and the skin around that eye was often swollen. The right side of her face and her right hand both twitched involuntarily, and her legs always felt restless.

"I was literally falling apart," Sue said in discouragement. Her long search for knowledgeable medical help had only revealed what she did not have and what treatments would not work. She still had no diagnosis other than chronic fatigue syndrome, and pharmaceutical treatments for that condition had proven intolerable so far. Left with a depleted savings account, Sue had to continue her search for healthcare on borrowed funds.

By Happenstance

"Then the most amazing thing happened," Sue said. That summer, Sue was trying to fill out financial paperwork in preparation for her divorce proceedings, but she was incapable of doing the math. "My math skills were at about a grade 2 level," Sue said as she explained her need for help.

As a result, she hired a woman to come to her home and do that work for her. One day while the woman was at Sue's home, she began to relate a story about a friend she knew who had Lyme disease. She told Sue that there were striking similarities between her symptoms and this friend's. She also asked Sue if she would like to talk to her friend about it, and Sue said that she would.

After Sue's helper left, Sue did some Internet research on Lyme disease where she found the Canadian Lyme Disease Foundation's website. The website listed 78 possible symptoms associated with Lyme disease, and Sue recognized 58 of them applied to her personally. "Even so, being a girl whose faith in the accuracy of the medical system was steadfast, I was still convinced that since my lab results were negative, I could not have Lyme disease," said Sue.

Shortly after this, the woman who had Lyme disease called Sue, and they spoke about the disease and her symptoms. "She told me about a doctor who came to the Island once a month to do Lyme clinics," Sue related. Encouraged, Sue made an appointment with this doctor. After carefully examining her and going over her medical history, he felt that it was likely that she was suffering from disseminated Lyme disease, and that it was affecting her brain. "Immediately, he ordered some more blood tests to see if I might have any co-infections that are often associated with Lyme. He [also] put me on a course of antibiotics."

With this newly discovered information, Sue returned to her general practitioner and told her what she had learned. Rather than being interested in Sue's information, the doctor responded sharply to Sue. "[She] was very upset that I had been out searching, once again, for the source of my illness without her referring me. She was not supportive of me taking antibiotics." Sadly, Sue's relationship with her general practitioner came under intense strain. Her doctor took issue with her taking antibiotics since Sue was not tolerating them very well.

Insurance Denial

During September of 2003, Sue's insurance company sent her a formal letter by courier stating that her long-term disability benefits had been terminated. "They advised [me] that in their opinion, I was now recovered from my leg surgery and back injuries. [Furthermore], since no formal testing had been done to measure my cognitive dysfunction, it was not considered a bar to my returning to my regular job; [consequently], further entitlement was denied."

Sue had 20 days to appeal this decision, and she did. However, while she was gathering the information required to do so, she stopped taking her antibiotics. "I stopped taking the antibiotics because I was so sick while I was on them. I needed to have as much strength as I could muster to get letters from the doctors I had seen and [gather] information to support my appeal. It was a horrible time."

During her appeal, Sue had been diagnosed with a probable case of Lyme disease, since the results of her latest tests had not come in yet. As a result, all of the other doctors who had seen her agreed with the psychologist's earlier diagnosis of chronic fatigue syndrome.

Despite Sue's medical consult letters and proof of disability, the insurance company denied her appeal advising that she did not "fit the profile for chronic fatigue syndrome." Sue said, "The decision letter skirted around the issue of chronic fatigue syndrome and said that the doctors did not know the reason why I was feeling the way I was. Since there was no reason, I was not considered disabled, and therefore, my claim was denied."

Interestingly, Sue's personal conversation with the insurance adjuster was far more revealing and sympathetic. "She said to me that during their review, they felt I probably did have Lyme disease, but that we had not gone down that path but rather the CFS path." The adjuster told Sue that she would reopen the claim if it was medically substantiated that Sue had Lyme disease.

At the time of the appeal denial, a number of doctor appointments were still lined up. Sue decided to keep these despite the denial, because she still had one last opportunity to appeal to the three doctors on the Medical Review Panel. She thought that these consultations might help her to present convincing medical evidence to that appeal board.

In October, Sue saw a psychiatrist, who felt certain that her problems were psychological in nature and suggested routine therapy. "Although I have been anxious," Sue said, "I have never felt depression. The neurocognitive studies showed that I was not depressed. I told the psychiatrist, but she replied that those tests are not always right."

Sue felt terribly humiliated by her assessment, and as she was leaving the psychiatrist's office, the doctor said, "I know exactly what you are going through. I have a cousin in Ireland who had exactly the same symptoms as [you]." What that had to do with anything, Sue did not know, but she never returned to this doctor. Incidentally, the psychiatrist's report stated that she felt Sue had "brain exhaustion"—an ambiguous assessment of no help to Sue's appeal efforts.

Following this encounter, Sue met with a rheumatologist. After his exam, he concluded that he did not know what was wrong with her. He did add, however, that he had seen other patients like her, who had become ill following a major surgery and who recovered two or three years later. He was also certain that her illness was "clearly neurological."

While waiting for the test results, Sue's skepticism about Lyme disease remained strong. "I felt that if I did have it, it would have shown up on my [earlier] Provincial lab tests." Sue was referred to an internal medicine specialist who had taken a few years away from his practice to participate in writing for the *Journal of Chronic Fatigue Syndrome*. When Sue consulted with him, he was once again practicing on the Island. He examined Sue and had no question that she suffered from chronic fatigue syndrome with severe cognitive deficit. He also felt that, although Lyme disease was rare, it was very likely the causative agent for her chronic fatigue syndrome.

Closing in

Sue's world was quickly closing in around her like a tightening noose. By December, new disabling symptoms were appearing at a frightening pace and presenting potentially dangerous threats to her. One of these symptoms included frequently occurring episodes of blackouts. She explained, "I [was] driving down the road and suddenly, I [did not] know where I was or what I was doing. It was as though I had been asleep for a split second and [woke] up suddenly. I became afraid to drive for fear I would have an accident." Sue reported these occurrences to her doctors, and they speculated that she might be experiencing small seizures.

As a result, Sue decided to limit her driving to necessary trips to doctors' appointments, prescription pick-ups, and grocery shopping. This single change of lifestyle brought to her attention the chasm that lay between her and good health. For an athlete who once spent a great deal of time outdoors and away from home, she was now limited to very few trips outside the house. Her world was shrinking in around her quickly.

Even within the confines of her own home, Sue realized there were simple things she was no longer capable of doing such as putting a meal together. "I had [decided] not to cook because I could no longer remember how to sequentially put a meal together. I could not follow recipes. The words did not make sense." Then, there were the potential dangers associated with short-term memory dysfunction. "I [forgot] that I had put something on to cook, and I [often left] the house with the oven or stove going."

Furthermore, her forgetfulness caused confusion and repetition of tasks already performed. "Once an avid reader, I could no longer read a novel and understand the meaning of the words on the page. If I set the book down, I could not remember what I had read the night before. Every night I picked up the same book and wondered how the bookmark was stuck into it when I hadn't even started the book yet! My life was like the movie, *Groundhog Day*."

Sue's memory became so bad that others could not help but notice its carry over into her social world. She explained, "I had a girlfriend come to visit from another town, and I stepped out of the house just after she arrived and completely forgot she was in the house. I left her in there, and it never occurred to me, as I puttered around outside, that I had company. [When] I had company, I [prepared] tea and goodies only to leave them in another room. It never occurred to me to serve them."

Inside her world of fleeting thoughts, she often alarmed herself by her own forgotten actions. One example of this occurred while trying to rearrange her bedroom furniture. "I [began] to change my room around and then left the room. A few minutes later, [I] returned to the room to become suddenly alarmed that my house had been broken into! I stood there and wondered why someone would make such a mess in my room. I didn't remember doing it," Sue said.

Positive Test Results

A bright light was cast into Sue's darkening world on December 24, 2003, when her Lyme disease Western blot results came back from a United States lab. Almost joyously

Sue explained, "My test results came back strongly positive for Lyme disease!" Sue's doctor immediately consulted with an infectious disease doctor who advised him to be skeptical over the report because "the lab results had far too many false positives to be credible evidence," and besides, "we do not have Lyme disease on the Island."

After the holidays passed, Sue was referred to another infectious disease specialist in February 2004. "I had been [forewarned] that I [might] be met with hostility and disbelief that I had Lyme disease. I was warned that for some reason, there were political issues around the Lyme disease diagnosis and that doctors were not willing to diagnose or treat since the treatment [involved] large doses of antibiotic therapy."

Despite her preconceptions, the meeting went well. The doctor performed a thorough exam and took an excellent history, treating Sue with deep respect and professional attentiveness. At the end of the exam, he told Sue that if she did not have Lyme disease right now, he was most certain that she had contracted it in the past. He also told her that he would use intravenous (IV) antibiotic therapy in Sue's particular case.

The doctor ordered a brain MRI that showed more lesions than were found ten months earlier. He also ordered a lumbar puncture to see if there might be additional evidence to support the Lyme disease diagnosis. Although this test did not add anything to further substantiate the diagnosis, the doctor installed a PICC (peripherally inserted central catheter) line through Sue's arm into her chest and started her on IV Rocephin therapy on May 12, 2004.

Intravenous Therapy

About that same time, Sue's final appeal to the Medical Review Panel on the mainland had been heard, and her disability claim was accepted. At last, hope had resurfaced with a vigorous gasp of life. It had been submerged for a long time—nearly two years since her leg surgery after which her first neurological problems appeared.

However, the fight was hardly over. Four days into her IV therapy, her pleural space started to fill with fluid, and the lower part of her lung collapsed. The infectious disease specialist explained to her that her lung dysfunction may have been part of a Herxheimer reaction to the bacterial kill-off initiated by the IV antibiotics. He told her that he had seen this happen around the heart before but never around the lung. Since Lyme disease was so complex, he could not rule it out as a cause of the problem.

As she was recovering from this setback, she developed an allergic reaction to Rocephin. Her resulting fever and blistering rash were treated in the emergency room at the local hospital. At this time, her doctor changed the IV antibiotic from Rocephin to penicillin, which she tolerated. Penicillin G was delivered to her system via an infusion pump—six million units every four hours.

During the next four weeks of therapy, Sue was ill and spent most of the time in bed. However, by the fourth week, she started to feel a resurgence of energy. By the 7th week, she was feeling even better. Her neurological symptoms and "crushing brain fatigue" still bothered her at times, but her overall energy level had significantly improved, and her joint pain had diminished notably.

Throughout the therapy, the hospital's IV team determined that Sue was not "reliable" to administer her own treatment at home. Instead, nurses came to her home every day. "There was no way that I could remember or figure out how to do the different things [involving] the pump and tubing every day. I [was] just too confused," Sue recalled.

On June 30, Sue finished her IV therapy and decided to hold off on oral antibiotics for a time to see how she fared after this stressful therapy. She happily maintained the increased level of energy produced by her therapy; however, her brain still functioned poorly allowing her only brief periods of mental clarity each morning. Sue still struggled with transient pain. Following her treatment, her parotid (salivary) gland in her face became painful and swollen. However, now that her doctor knew the cause of her symptoms, they were treated not as isolated cases of disease, but as complex and transient symptoms of chronic Lyme disease.

Over her Shoulder

Sue does not look over her shoulder longingly at what she used to be or what she used to enjoy. She doesn't need to do that to know what she has lost in her social, professional, and personal worlds. "Those losses encompass having to essentially sever myself from the community, my friends, from activities, and from any kind of work. I had to cut myself off from people and life as a means of survival just so that I could function at a low level," Sue said.

She has faith only that things "will get better" and her athlete's resolve drives her to achieve greater progress toward regaining some of her former good health. The knowledge she has learned about Lyme disease has helped her to understand the disease progression as she experienced it.

She is also grateful for one key person about whom she makes this admission. "Had I not hired that lady to do my [financial] books, I would probably still be very ill to this day and not know what was causing my illness." Until the medical community more skillfully recognizes the early clinical presentations of Lyme disease, it will continue to fall upon the shoulders of the ill to find those scarce sources of knowledgeable medical help. At present, this connection of patient with knowledgeable physician is more often than not, facilitated through the unexpected voice of a caring friend or even an acquaintance as in Sue's case.

Sue has also discovered another element to her medical history. "Lyme disease often lays quietly in the system until the immune system is run down or after an accident, surgery, or childbirth [experience]...some type of [stress or trauma] to the body. This is exactly what happened in my case. I would never have suspected something like this because I did not question that the testing methods used by our medical system were not absolute," she said.

Sue learned that relying solely on laboratory tests, incorrectly employing those tests, and stringently interpreting the results outside the context of the entire clinical picture has often resulted in many Lyme disease patients losing years of valuable treatment time. Meanwhile, widely disseminated bacterial infection and extensive neurological damage may occur as evidenced in Sue Ferguson's case history.

Sue observed, "Lyme disease is supposed to be a clinical diagnosis, yet the doctors seem to rely on laboratory testing as the sole method of making the diagnosis. The treatment for Lyme disease seems to be highly controversial. IV therapy seems to be the treatment of choice for central nervous system Lyme disease, but apparently, it has to be ordered by an infectious disease doctor. Very few infectious disease doctors will do this."

Caring for Self

Out of necessity, Sue realized that she had to make lifestyle changes in order to deal with her illness. "I had to take everything down a notch with my lifestyle, then I had to drop it more notches and more notches. I live a much slower pace which is a lot healthier for anyone. I never try to push through exhaustion anymore. I have learned that if I feel it coming on, I rest. That rest means I am able to function the next day."

Sue created boundaries to protect herself, and she had become stronger because of them. One of those boundaries included being selective about her surroundings because stress and negativity drained her of precious energy. "Stress can take me down faster than anything physical. I learned to define the stresses [because] I cannot be around negative people or in negative situations."

This called for more assertive communication with others. "I've learned to be upfront with people and tell them I can't have guests for more than an hour. I can't have weekend company. Before, I always put myself last and others first. Now I care for myself." Sue realized quickly that she had to take control of her life if she wanted to enjoy even a small ration of good health.

Now she takes pleasure in the simple joys of life. "I just sit and enjoy the weather. If I go for a walk with friends, we can sit on a log and just enjoy that time in silence. We don't always have to be running in life." For perhaps the first time in her life, the athlete in her had learned the value of "being still."

Two Years Later

In August 2004, two years after she first became symptomatic, Sue spoke of her future and said, "We will just have to wait and see how this [treatment] goes. At this time in my life, I can't imagine ever going back to claims adjudication in the trauma unit. I can't imagine what I would do for employment because of the severe short-term memory problems and fatigue that challenge me every day."

Sue has spoken to others who have recovered from Lyme disease and returned to work. She hangs on to a similar hope for herself. "I hope this treatment will work, and I will get my brain and some energy back." To Sue, Lyme disease is one of the most formidable foes that exists in the realm of infectious diseases. "It takes [away] a person's ability to function physically but also takes [away] the ability to function mentally. I can't imagine what other disease renders a person as disabled as this."

Those who deal with chronic Lyme disease clearly understand Sue's sentiments. With the help of friendships she has made through Lyme support societies, Sue is encouraged to push on in the greatest race of her life, the contest for her mind and soul. Sue summed it up this way, "I have never stopped believing that this is just a short pause in the flow of my life, and that I will get better. What is most important to me is that I know, in my heart, I will be back on my bikes, and I will climb again as those are the things I am passionate about."

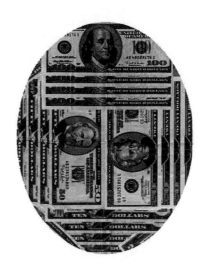

The Money Lender

"Gold that buys health can never be ill spent."
—*John Webster*

Michael Daniels made it his business to know the value of the dollar. As a successful vice president of a large bank in California, he enjoyed the every day challenges of the financial world. He knew the many lucrative uses of money and skillfully made it a banker's gainful servant.

Life was fast-paced, and work days were long as Mike supervised 30 West Coast branch managers and their lending operations. Traveling frequently to and from these affiliated offices, he consulted with the managers, taught classes on lending, and trained key bank personnel. At the main office, he often met with customers, approved loan applications, and also assisted the area manager with the business performances of the entire group of branches.

He earned a very good reputation with the bank and among his business associates. Mike recalled, "I was pretty young, at the top of my game, and [I] was doing the things that I needed to do to be successful. I did work very hard, though, and really enjoyed it. I also enjoyed the limelight of the success that I was having." An avid golfer, Mike played about twice a week with business associates. "It was a good way to make new friends as [I] came into a new area with the bank," he explained.

He seemed equally successful in his social world. "I played on a very competitive softball team. We were undefeated, at one point, for almost two years in a very competitive environment," Mike said. In civic affairs, Mike took a very active role. He served as treasurer of the local Kiwanis club and was active on various committees, and also, in the Chamber of Commerce. "My wife and I had a very active social life while we were living there, and we made a lot of friends," he said.

In the winter of 1985, Mike accepted a job transfer, a promotion to a bank in Los Gatos, California. The merger of the main office with Los Gatos was part of a large consolidation effort organized by the bank. Instead of being offered a manager's position with one of the 30 branch offices, Mike was given an opportunity to join the present merger. "I was very fortunate, at the time, to get to go [to Los Gatos]," he reflected.

Los Gatos was an upscale bedroom community located on Highway 17 between San Jose and Santa Cruz. Its ideal location brought in heavy tourism and attracted wealthy retirees and other professionals with money and leisure time to spare. At the time of Mike's transfer, he envisioned a happy and prosperous life for himself, his wife, *Rebecca*, and his children.

Though grateful for the transfer invitation, Mike was, in actuality, one of the bank's top performers in the West

Coast region. He had been recognized and rewarded by the bank in all the typical ways: stock options, stock awards, bonuses, trips, and gifts. Whenever top executive banking guests were being wined and dined, Mike played an active role as business host during these visits. Without a doubt, Mike was enjoying the pinnacle of career success.

At thirty-six years of age, Mike basked in good health and bountiful energy. "At the time, I felt pretty much bulletproof," he said. He needed no other doctor than the sun, fresh air, and a competitive game of softball. The new locality and its surrounding areas offered all those things and more: ball parks, golf courses, nearby forests, lakes, and state parks.

It was a paradise of sporting pleasure, and he took advantage of it by playing weekly softball games, golfing, and taking family camping trips each summer. "I also loved to take care of the yard around the house. I mowed the whole 2 ½ acres every week during the spring and fall seasons. I [rode] my riding mower, and then [I would] weed eat around all 150 oak trees every week in shorts and sandals," he explained.

In his upscale neighborhood of heavily wooded lots, it was very common to observe abundant numbers of deer foraging for food, and in the process, destroying property and decorative garden and landscaping plants. They had become a real nuisance to people like Mike, who took pride in the presentation of his yard. "There would always be ten to twenty deer on our property every day [without fail]," he said. Other wildlife such as squirrels, rabbits, raccoons, and skunks flourished there along with an occasional wild turkey and fox.

Something else thrived there too—ticks. "I never noticed the ticks, [but] we had a dog that my [family] used to pull ticks off of [frequently]." Personally, Mike was terribly repulsed by ticks and would not even look at them, but he has since wondered about his exposure to them while working in his yard.

First Symptoms

Barely two weeks had passed since Mike's relocation when he became terribly sick. For the next three weeks, he experienced diarrhea, nausea, sweats, chills, and weight loss. Recalling this aggressive sickness, he said, "I was afraid that I had some very serious illness and that I was dying. Because of that fear, I didn't go to the doctor for quite a while." Mike's father finally convinced him to consult with a medical professional, if for no other reason than to squelch the worries of the family. He complied, and his blood was drawn for testing.

After examining the resulting test report, the physician diagnosed Mike with giardiasis. This disease is caused by intestinal protozoa and is usually associated with drinking contaminated water. Symptoms include notable diarrhea, and diagnosis is most often made by microscopic visualization of the organism in stool samples.

"I never did understand how I could have obtained giardia. I did not drink any contaminated water that I knew of. [Previously] I drank only treated water; [now] I drink from our well, usually. It wasn't treated, but it was from a well that was 400 feet [deep]. That water had been tested at the time that they dug the well, and it was not contaminated. I always wondered how I could have possibly gotten giardia. Even at the time, I had no reason to think that it was anything else," Mike related.

Treated with a short course of strong antibiotics, his symptoms subsided within a couple of days. He felt well again and went back to work. He thought that was the end of the story. After about one year, however, Mike gradually began to experience soreness in his right hip. Tylenol seemed to take care of most of the discomfort at that point in time. This was the same hip that he had broken in a motorcycle accident when he was 18 years of age. Naturally, he wondered if there was a connection between that earlier injury and his current, arthritic-type of pain.

Mike never noticed a sudden onset of this new hip pain. It just crept up on him. When the pain kept recurring and additional joints began to ache, he went to see his family doctor. "He could not come up with any reason for these problems. [However], he prescribed an anti-inflammatory medication and enough pain medicine so that I would have one [prescription pain reliever] when I really needed it," Mike explained.

By seeming coincidence, Mike also began experiencing visual problems. One morning as he woke and looked around him, the vision through his right eye seemed to have a smoky ring around it. He immediately went to an ophthalmologist, who diagnosed him with iritis (inflammation of the iris, the colored portion of the eye) along with a subsequent rare form of glaucoma. The ophthalmologist prescribed some eye drops for Mike and told him that in a week or so, his symptoms would clear up and go away, but they did not.

Eventually, Mike had surgery on his eye to relieve the pressure from fluid that had built up inside. A surgical opening functioned well for a while, draining any excess ocular fluid. In time, however, the surgical opening grew shut, and his eye symptoms reappeared. He went back to a regimen of applying four to five different eye drops a day for relief of his glaucoma.

Frustrated that neither his vision problem nor his hip pain had subsided, he said, "Over the next ten years, both of these problems became more and more troublesome. My hip pain became not only worse, but it spread to my other joints. It moved to my left hip, then to almost every joint in my body. The various medications for inflammation and pain became less effective as well [as did] the eye drops for my glaucoma."

A Priceless Advocate

Mike's wife, Rebecca, took a very supportive role during this time. She relentlessly poured over medical books, newspaper articles, searched the Internet, and gleaned ideas from others. Frequently, she took her ideas to their family doctor, asking for his professional opinion. "During the times [when] I was seeing different doctors, if she was not happy with my descriptions of my last doctor's appointment, she would insist on going with me to the next one," Mike said.

Having such a loyal advocate was priceless, especially when Mike felt depleted of energy and motivation. Driven by her love and concern for him, Rebecca went to many of Mike's appointments with him and took a prominent speaking role at these consultations. She had done the research beforehand and prepared well for each of these visits. Furthermore, she was well acquainted with Mike's medical history so that she knew what worked, what didn't, and how he was feeling as a result. He noted, "Almost every new thing we tried, or new idea we came up with, was because of her. I was feeling so bad and getting so discouraged that sometimes I just [wasn't] able to care."

He and Rebecca continued their search for a diagnosis; and in the meantime, Mike endured the pains associated with his symptoms. He was no stranger to pain or suffering, he said. He recalled surviving childhood surgeries—and later reconstructive surgery—and a long rehabilitation period after a motorcycle wreck that broke most of the bones in his body. With these painful experiences behind him, he felt certain that he had the kind of endurance needed to face his present circumstances. However, he admitted that he was growing tired of not feeling well, and apparently so were others.

Nothing Personal

Mike knew that his job performance at the bank was suffering and that he had to do something quickly about his advancing illness. He was in pain most of the time and was so fatigued that he could hardly make it through the day. "This developed over a long period of time—years. My slide down took a pretty long time as well, but after a certain point, it went quickly. The last two-three years were the worst."

In the corporate world, no one is irreplaceable. This fact is especially pronounced in the banking industry where an employee is an investment for which a return is expected. If an employee cannot perform this role for any reason, a termination is in order. It is purely business, "nothing personal" as the rhetoric goes.

Nevertheless, the termination of a chronically ill employee, such as Mike, can be an extremely sensitive matter in light of current discrimination laws. Carefully orchestrated circumstances are sometimes designed to lay the foundation for a legal, face-saving termination. Mike suspected that he was being placed into such circumstances when he was assigned to duties that were nearly impossible for him to perform.

"They gave me four branches to manage. I had been given a particularly growing area, so the goals were huge. The results weren't. While I was getting more and more ill, the results of these four units were going south quickly," Mike said. If he wanted to save his job, he had to regain his health.   Perhaps a specialist could help?

The Rheumatologist

"After I had been seeing my family doctor for several years, with the problems getting more and more severe, she referred me to a rheumatologist [who] worked with me for several months into years. At first, she thought I had ankylosing spondylitis (a progressive rheumatic disorder), [and] she treated me as if I had that for quite a while. She also thought, at one point, that I might have had hepatitis or something like that because of the pain."

He was treated by this specialist for years for various diseases that she thought he might have contracted. "I don't think anything that she prescribed made me feel worse. Nothing really made me feel better, though," Mike said. Actually, the most helpful prescription he received from her was a pain reliever for arthralgia.

In 2000, Mike's symptoms dramatically worsened, and so, he took a 30 day sick leave from work. When he returned to work again, he felt more rested and even more determined to help his mini-group of branches meet their financial goals. He explained, "I actually called in all the markers that I had ever made. I single-handedly brought in enough business for the four stores to turn around and start hitting their goals for one quarter. Unfortunately, the results for the prior period were too much to overcome. At the same time, my company had been bought out by another company from the South. Everyone who had come from my former company was marked. One day, most of us got it."

In prior years, Mike had always been able to escape termination by merit of his position within the company. This time was very different. "At the time, the corporate [explanation] was that my job had been eliminated due to the merger of my company with another bank." However, Mike felt certain that he lost his job because his illness prohibited him from being "up to my former self." This ended 25 years of service with the bank.

Retiring at 54 years of age, even with a generous severance package of 18 months at full pay, was not a viable option for Mike and his family. He wanted to work, but he was really too ill to perform steadily at a job. Consequently, six months passed before he was feeling well enough to even look for another job.

A Growing Hunch

The exhaustion Mike felt after he lost his job was immobilizing. He said, "I needed to find work, but [I] didn't feel like doing anything." Rebecca did some of the leg work for him, talking to everyone she knew who had experiences with mysterious or undiagnosed illnesses. "Around that time, my wife had come across an article or some other information about Lyme [disease]. [She] was thinking that it could possibly be what I had because [I] did have some of the [same] symptoms [she read about], but also, because [the disease] was new, and no one had ever come across it before."

Every time the Daniels consulted with a doctor, Rebecca raised the suggestion that perhaps Mike suffered from Lyme disease. "It became something she was talking about more and more because there were fewer and fewer [viable] possibilities. No [physician] was coming up with anything else," Mike explained. In each case, the doctor dismissed Rebecca's suggestion, and Mike was beginning to wonder if anyone had any knowledge of the illness. It did not appear so.

Continuing their search for knowledgeable medical advice, Mike and Rebecca introduced the idea of Lyme disease to the rheumatologist and, also, to their family doctor at their next appointment. Mike observed that both doctors expressed serious doubts about the disease in general, and so they were unwilling to offer professional advice on this disease. "My family doctor, an old friend, had told me privately that he had been hearing a lot about that disease [in 2001], but that he didn't understand it [and] could not see how [my illness] could possibly be anything like that."

However, after years of inaccurate diagnoses and ineffective treatments, the family doctor and the rheumatologist agreed to facilitate Mike's out-patient admission to a research hospital at the University of San Francisco. Furthermore, Mike's doctor suggested that he and Rebecca ask about Lyme disease when they were there for diagnostic testing.

At the hospital, Mike was led through a battery of tests. With every doctor or technician he encountered, he or Rebecca asked whether his illness could be Lyme disease. The responses that they received to that suggestion appeared oddly absent of medical curiosity, especially for a research hospital. "No one there would even admit to the possibility that I might have it. I don't even know if they had ever heard of it," Mike recalled.

Regardless, Mike proceeded through a full day of diagnostic testing which included a comprehensive blood panel. "I didn't see one specialist. After I was finished, I was told that the doctors from that department were going to review the results and discuss it at their general department meeting to compare notes and thoughts and [to] see if anything productive came of it. Well, apparently, nothing did."

Despite the extensive testing, no diagnostic conclusions were drawn. One suggestion was made that seemed more of an insult than medical advice. Mike said, "They didn't know what I had but [suggested that] maybe my pain was imagined and that perhaps I just had a virus or something."

This was not the first time that this type of medical opinion had been suggested to him. "The thing that I was hearing the most was that it must have been some form of an imagined pain or phantom pain with possibly the nerve ends damaged or something. The feeling of this [indescribable] 'fever' that I had, [was explained as] possibly some form of depression and on and on." Frustrated and discouraged, Mike returned home to resume his existing therapy with eye drops and pain relievers.

After Dinner Advice

Mike realized that his illness had become publicly known in the community. "People were talking all over town about me and how sick I was. [They] also had heard that I had gone to San Francisco to meet with some pretty high level specialists to see what I might have. So everyone was talking about everything. Of course, there were other prominent people in town who had been diagnosed with Lyme [disease]. One of them was a lady [friend of ours]," Mike said.

Their friend had recently tested positive for Lyme disease and was undergoing treatment when Mike and Rebecca met up with her at a dinner function. The dinner was held in honor of a gentleman who was just hired for a position that Mike wanted—executive director of a certain hospital foundation. Having once been president of a hospital foundation, Mike thought he had a good chance at securing this job. After he learned that he lost the position to his friend, he thought that perhaps his publicly known illness might have been a large factor in that outcome.

Despite the circumstances, Mike was happy to attend the dinner in his friend's honor. Many prominent people from the community were present, and as Mike and Rebecca mingled among them, they engaged in a number of private conversations. The topic seemed to revolve frequently around Mike's health and his recent trip to San Francisco. "People were asking me about my trip and [whether or not] I had mentioned Lyme disease [while at the hospital]," he said.

While Mike was conversing, Rebecca was coincidentally having her own conversation with the woman who was being treated for Lyme disease. As she listened to the description of her symptoms, there was a ring of familiarity to it. The more Rebecca listened to their friend's experience, the more convinced she became that this disease might be the cause of Mike's debilitating symptoms.

When they returned home after the dinner, Mike and Rebecca discussed the evening's conversations that they had shared with friends. When the topic of their friend's Lyme disease was raised, Rebecca told Mike that she had an informative conversation with her about it, and she proceeded to tell him what she had learned. Noting a possible source of medical help, Rebecca also obtained the name of the neurologist who was treating their friend. Now, both Mike and Rebecca had more reason to believe that perhaps their physicians had overlooked a very likely cause for his disabling ailments.

A Knowledgeable Source

With renewed hope, Mike called the neurologist's office to make an appointment. The doctor agreed to see him, but informed him that she was no longer taking new patients with Lyme disease. "At that time, she was the only doctor that I knew of [who] was treating Lyme disease patients," Mike said. He hoped the doctor would reconsider and take his case if he really did have the infection.

Undeterred, Mike went to his appointment and

quickly developed a positive rapport with the doctor, even discovering they had friends in common. Once past the initial niceties of their introduction, the doctor spoke to him in general terms and shared basic facts about Lyme disease with him. Ultimately, though, she agreed to provide the test kits to Mike so that he could have his blood tested for Lyme disease. Eager to have these tests done, he was willing to pay the out-of-pocket costs. "My insurance would not cover the tests, so [I] had to take care of obtaining the kits, going to the lab, and getting the results back to the doctor [myself]," Mike recalled.

Various tests were performed including a Western blot, and the results of those tests were positive for Lyme disease. Certain now of the origin of his painful symptoms, he said, "I had a very serious case of Lyme [disease], and [I] had it for a long time." Finally, the correlation was clearly made between his initial flu-like symptoms, his hip pain, vision problems, his widespread myalgias, and other troubling symptoms. Mike understood, finally, that all of these symptoms originated from a common cause and that he had been living with chronic Lyme disease for the past 16 years.

Rheumatologist's Reaction

Mike was curious to know what his rheumatologist would say about his Lyme disease test results, so he took them to her on one of his many follow-up visits. "She insisted that I didn't have it every time that I saw her. I could never figure that one out. Every time I spoke to her about this, that was her response, and yet, nothing she had done had helped me at all," Mike said.

This marked a definite turning point in their doctor-patient relationship. Her refusal to acknowledge the positive test results or the new doctor's diagnosis of Lyme disease made any further consultations with her nonproductive. In addition, she also began to deny Mike refills of his prescription pain medication. Mike felt her unspoken dismissal as he faced a new dilemma. "I was in so much pain at that time [that] I didn't know what I was going to do," Mike recalled.

That was the last time Mike went to see the rheumatologist. "She realized that she could not help me, and she did not understand the disease that I had, [and yet she knew] another doctor had been able to diagnose me correctly," Mike said. From then on, he relied upon the help of the neurologist who had diagnosed him.

Treatment Begins

The first thing that the neurologist did was to offer Mike some printed information on Lyme disease, since he had virtually no knowledge of his illness. She explained the progression of the disease and how, in his case, the disease had reached a widely disseminated state affecting many body systems. She advised him about chronic Lyme disease and about what he might expect from the recommended antibiotic protocol. "She also suggested that I might never be totally over the disease, but that as long as we could reach a place where [I] could live comfortably—a sort of baseline spot—then that might be all right," remembered Mike.

Informed of the possible treatment limitations, the neurologist prescribed an aggressive intravenous antibiotic therapy for Mike. A peripherally inserted central catheter (PICC line) was inserted into a large vein near the inside of his elbow and threaded up into his chest cavity. For the next several months, Mike administered the prescribed antibiotics into the PICC line himself at home. "I gave myself the hypo syringes two or three times a day, and I [went] into the hospital weekly to get the PICC line cleaned out," Mike recalled. When he did so, he also picked up his next week's supply of medicine and stored it at home in his refrigerator. Throughout the intravenous therapy, the doctor changed the antibiotic or adjusted the dosage to meet Mike's needs. As bacterial die-off occurred, he experienced Herxheimer-like reactions or flares in symptoms. "I just felt terrible. I felt like my whole body had a fever...like my body was inflamed," he explained. During those times, Mike experienced a total lack of energy. His eye flared up, muscles ached, and pain radiated from all areas of his body.

A Daunting Search

Despite his disease flares, he could tell that he was regaining a measure of health. He finally felt strong enough to look for another job, yet the thought of searching was daunting. "That was one of the hardest things that I had ever done. All of the people and companies that I thought I would be able to get a job with, or go to work for, did not want to hire me because they knew I had been sick," Mike said.

His search for work was met by resistance from an unexpected source—his friends. Some of these friends were individuals who were indebted to Mike for his prior acts of kindness towards them. "My (former) friends looked the other way when I tried to convince them that I was no longer ill [and] was ready to go back to work and really, really, really needed the job. Several of those people had been helped in very big ways by me when they had needed help in prior years," Mike recalled.

These experiences occurred over a period of several months, but Mike drew strength from within. "I am a very strong person. I have gotten over many, many, hard times and experiences in my life." Despite his personal armor, even Mike had his moments of despair. "Then one day, when I was driving down the road, having been just given the shove out the door again, I called my 84-year-old father and broke down. I have never felt as bad in my life as I did that day. He felt worse. He couldn't help the son that he had always been able to help any time he was ever asked."

Starting Over

In 2002, Mike finally secured a new job with a regional bank as a conventional business loan underwriter. "When I started, I wasn't sure that I would be able to do it, but I was. I had to pretty much start over. I have been doing underwriting for large commercial business loans. I hadn't really done that for over ten years, and some of what I do, I had never done before."

Since then, Mike has performed well in his new position, but not without challenges. Admittedly, Lyme disease affected his cognitive powers. "My short term memory is not good at all. That is really bad in my job. Many of the things that we do, do not have a manual or [written] instruction. I forget how to do new things all of the time. I try to write them down as soon as I learn them, but that's not always possible."

That is also the case when it comes to routine conversations at the workplace. Mike said, "Sometimes people will tell me something, [or] a customer, or one of the branches, or other employees. If I don't write it down, there is a good chance that I will forget it."

Another cognitive problem that developed from Mike's case of Lyme disease was dyslexia. "Numbers don't always register in my brain correctly. I have always been very good at mathematics and computations. I now do financial spreads and other financial analyses all of the time for many hours a day. I very often put down numbers backwards or somehow invert them or otherwise put them out of order. When I do that, it will [sometimes] take me hours to find. I have to find it, because financial analysis involves money, a lot of money," Mike explained.

Naturally, Mike is guarded against sharing information about his health with his employer. "I have had a concern since I began my employment here, that if the company knew that I was experiencing this difficulty, they might decide that they don't want to run the risk of me making a big mistake. I do make mistakes, but fortunately, so does everyone else. Also, I work very hard at correcting my errors, and [I] usually find them."

During times when he experiences disease flares, he has taken extraordinary care to perform well on the job. "Sometimes, I don't feel well. I don't know for sure, but it feels exactly like when I was the sickest. I am not as quick. I make more errors, and I don't interact very well with other employees. No one knows why I am acting different, but I do," he said.

Mike works very hard at his job, burning the midnight oil in order to maintain top performance and to protect his job. "As a result of my hard work and long, long, long hours, I have been the top producing underwriter at this large loan production center for the previous six consecutive quarters. I have worked here for six quarters plus one half. It took me the first half quarter to learn what I was doing."

In July of 2004, Mike was informed that he was the highest ranked employee at the center. Explaining, he said, "The ranking is determined by production plus many other factors, including teamwork, helping other employees, support of management, and cooperation." Certainly, it could be said that Mike Lawrence has gained the upper hand over his illness. He has recovered about 80% of his former good health and has found ways to deal with his weaknesses.

Chronic Lyme disease has also curbed Mike's participation in business meetings on the golf course. "I do not play golf at all anymore. My joints are too painful to do anything very physical," Mike said. While his business associates play golf twice a month, he must decline their invitations. "Since I can't golf, I don't get that opportunity to spend time with the decision makers who are out with the guys on the golf course. I have not disclosed to them why I don't play golf other than to say that I have bad joints. I know that they wonder what is wrong with me," he related.

Now more than ever, Mike knows that he must continue his efforts to keep his job. He sold his former large home and relocated a little closer to work. As empty nesters, Mike and Rebecca decided to downsize their residence in exchange for affordability, convenience, and less maintenance. "The home is less than two years old and is beautiful. We were able to put a pretty good down payment on it, but if I lost this job, we would be bankrupt." Mike understands the fragility of personal finances and how this house of cards stands precariously upon one's ability to remain steadily employed.

Employment Issues

Though Mike successfully protected his medical privacy on the job, he noted the disparity between his past and present perception of self. He said, "I think everyone knows what the prejudice is against employees who are ill. I will say that it is amazing how different it is to go from one of the people that the employees and everyone else always looked up to, and was envious of, to one that everyone feels badly for. Don't be mistaken, I am not really perceived by everyone here as a person [who] is somehow very sick. I work hard, long hours and produce more than anybody."

Having worked in both managerial and non-managerial employee positions, Mike has come to realize the serious issues surrounding chronically ill employees. "As a part of management in the past, the biggest problem with sick people is that they are not reliable. You don't know if they are going to show up for work," he noted. Certainly, if a job applicant is challenged on a daily basis with an ongoing illness, and yet this person is qualified and able to perform the daily duties for which he or she has applied, then it would be discriminatory not to hire that person. However, on the flip side, Mike noted that sometimes a chronically ill employee will resort to claiming all of his or her available sick day benefits prematurely, and, in the end, may quit or be terminated as a result. There is great frustration for both parties in this case.

Mike experienced this himself. "With my former employer, I could not believe it when I used up all of my saved up sick leave—even my long-term sick leave. When I had to take a month off because I was too sick to work, I was so humiliated. I had to do it, though, because even though I could actually bring myself in to work, I could not do the activities that it took to be successful on the job. How does a person sell financial services to high level customers or help other employees, [from] four whole branches, sell them as well? [Plus I had to] conduct training, staff meetings, and meet with customers. It was impossible," Mike recalled.

Keep Getting up!

Since Mike's experience with Lyme disease, many more cases of the disease have been reported where he lives. In fact, California is now recognized to have many endemic counties for Lyme disease. According to the Centers for Disease Control and Prevention (CDC), a county in which Lyme disease is endemic is one where at least two confirmed cases have been previously acquired or where established populations of a known tick vector are infected with B. burgdorferi. Mike said, "It has become quite a problem in the area. Increasing numbers of people are becoming sick, and more doctors who are willing to treat it are moving into the area."

Though not the first case on record, Mike certainly contracted Lyme disease at a time when the county medical community did not recognize the scope of the disease. Now, almost two decades later, Mike has found some humor in the way he endured it. "My wife and I have [jokingly] said over the past few years, that if someone were to write my epitaph now, it should read, "He kept getting up."

Having faced numerous personal trials in the past, Mike has made "keep getting up" his motto in life. "You can't let these things get you down," he said. His motto spurs him on like a prize fighter, and fight he must. Living with a constant level of pain frequently alters his moods. "I was always in a good mood, which is one of my biggest problems now. I am not happy all of the time," he noted.

This is a common challenge for chronic Lyme disease patients. Mike candidly explained, "I think that the one [thing] everyone, who has ever had it, mentions is the problems in trying to deal with it all. You don't hear it mentioned often about the emotional aspect of this illness. It is very depressing. When a person has been very active, very successful, and very healthy—[and] suddenly or slowly, loses [his] ability to enjoy life anymore—it is very hard to take. When you realize this isn't like a cold or the flu, that you are never going to be the same again, you almost don't want to be what you have become. It does take a while to get over that."

Mike faced these issues realistically, and in spite of the physical and emotional challenges chronic Lyme disease poses, he has risen above it. He has worked for his present employer for two years with a minimum of sick days. "I have been very successful in my new position. [However,] I do have some very difficult days," Mike said.

Family support was another important factor in

Mike's ability to endure the chronic nature of his illness. Fondly, he expressed gratitude to his wife and partner of over 30 years. "I do have a beautiful wife, who has been with me through everything that has ever happened to me. I have two beautiful children, who have never been anything but the most beautiful kids in the world. My parents, who are in their 80's, still have most of their health and are doing pretty well."

The Price of Change

Mike and his family understand, as only patient and caregivers can, that when someone in the family is seriously ill, everyone in the family "has to take the medicine," as Mike puts it. Everyone experienced the humbling effects of his unemployment and the resulting social status changes. Mike recalled, "When I was the community banker, I was one of the more prominent people in the community. I knew everyone, and everyone seemed to know me. It was always nice. We were invited to the best events. That was nice for the kids. They had a certain prestige that they lost when I became ill and then lost my job. They have handled it fantastically, but it was not easy for them, I'm sure."

Gone are the days of his indefatigable volunteerism and prestigious club memberships. The generous donations of time he gave to the Chamber of Commerce, Rotary Club, Hospital Foundation, Rodeo, Centennial Celebration, Community Symphony, and merchant-consumer events all seem to be simply part of his personal history now. When one lives in the fast lane, as Mike had for many years, and then by necessity must make a long pit stop, the race goes on regardless.

This was quite evident in what happened to Mike and Rebecca when they were members of the elite Porsche Touring Association. "It was a small club of Porsche owners with membership by invitation only," Mike said. Twice each year, the 20 member club would organize a road trip in their Porsche vehicles. The food and accommodations were always first class, and the association was light and humorously entertaining. The trips themselves were somewhere within a two day driving distance from Los Gatos, and the drive was beautiful.

Mike noted that his participation in such clubs was just as important as his performance at work. It was a privileged participation, but also an expected way of life in that stratum of society. "We were part of the club for several years until my health and our finances would no longer allow us to enjoy the excursions. We were pretty close friends with almost all of the members of that group. They were the same people we would see at Rotary, the Chamber of Commerce, and on, and on. We are really no longer friends with any of those people [now]." The raw reality is that life goes on. Mike's former colleagues still go on their road trips and do all the things they used to do, but they do it without him.

At his present job, Mike has built new friendships, but for the most part, he and Rebecca have gone back to more enduring relationships. "Today, we have a few of our old friends, but almost none of the friends from the period when we were 'on top' are still friends today. We have pretty much gone back to our old [lives] and a few friends who we have met along the way who are really special."

His successes on the job have helped him regain his self-esteem and confidence. "I have been able to obtain the job that I currently have, and I am doing very well at performing as well as I think that I can." Even with all these assets, Mike still relies on one more thing, "As I said, just keep getting up. Don't let it get you down...and pray a lot, a whole lot—prayers of thanks. It always works."

Still, there are times when Mike sits quietly at his desk and indulges in a moment of meandering thought—

"How would it feel to feel normal like all of these people? To just feel normal?"

Medicine Chest

Nearly 20 years after Mike became infected with Lyme disease and three years after starting successful treatment, Mike maintains his current level of health with the help of various medications. "I am weaning myself off the antibiotic now. [I am] going to try it without them for a while." He still takes four different eye drops for frequent glaucoma flare-ups, Celebrex for joint pain, and Provigil for fatigue. Occasionally, he will also take additional prescription pain relievers when the need arises.

Naturally, he would like to regain a greater measure of his former good health, but looking back over two decades of chronic illness, he is satisfied with where he is today. With gratitude he concluded, "Compared to how I felt prior to treatment, I feel very fortunate."

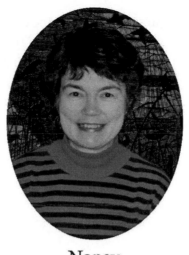

Nancy

The Spirit to Climb

"If a man constantly aspires, is he not elevated?"
—*Henry David Thoreau*

t was spring of 1996, and a gorgeous day had dawned on Mt. Hood, Oregon's tallest mountain. Created from alternating layers of lava flows, ash, and other volcanic debris, it rises to a height of 11,237 feet, making it an alluring climb for a trained mountaineer like 52-year-old Nancy Oace. As part of a 12 member climbing party, Nancy started her ascent at 1:00 a.m. on the east side of Mt. Hood, winding her way around it to the south side summit on the Sunshine route.

Roped to her nearest partners, Nancy cautiously negotiated the mountain's steep sides and deep, glacier crevasses with the aid of her ice axe. After winding around to the south side, she encountered the steepest part of the route.

At this point, she jammed her axe above and in front of her. Then she could use it to support the weight of her body as she pulled herself up to locate the next secure foothold. With her feet in place again and hands free to remove the axe, she repeated this technique as she slowly advanced toward the summit.

It was nearly noon, and the sun sprayed its blinding light over the snowy cap of Mt. Hood. Throughout the climb, Nancy had been breathing with her mouth open, and the reflection of the sun burned the roof of her mouth. Despite this, she felt exhilarated. "I felt very strong and confident during this part of the climb, and [I] was thankful that my energy was excellent," Nancy said.

Reaching the summit at 1:00 p.m., Nancy took a good, long gaze at the region from this glorious height. She saw a distant city and much of northeastern Oregon. It was simply awe-inspiring. She recalled, "It was a very powerful feeling when I reached the top of the mountain. People [who were] climbing up looked like ants, and the mountain that looked small from down below was, in reality, a very vast area."

Though trained professionally for this climb as a member of the Mazama Club, Nancy credited two other factors for her athletic feats: her propensity for endurance, which first came to her notice when she started climbing, and the learned qualities of patience and perseverance. Recalling her childhood when these traits were being developed, she said, "I had asthma and allergies as a child, and I got sick a lot. I also had rheumatic fever when I was seven which took several months to get over. These things strengthened me and gave me the will to overcome and be victorious." Little did she realize just how useful those qualities would become to her and how she would need them as she faced the greatest health challenge of her life.

The Pivotal Event

One Saturday in May of 1998, when Nancy was training for the upcoming climbing season, she decided to do some hiking on Franklin Ridge in Oregon's Columbia River Gorge. The following day, she also hiked the Elk-King traverse in the Coast Range. It seemed to be a routine exercise, but in actuality, it was a weekend that changed her life physically and spiritually.

On the following Tuesday, as she was bathing, she noticed a dark spot on the back of her left arm. Scrubbing did not remove it, so she put her glasses on and repulsively discovered that it was an attached tick. Nancy learned about the dangers of ticks in the Mazama Club, and she had always been very careful, but this one slipped by her immediate notice.

Around the tick was a circle of red, inflamed skin one and a half inches in diameter. She also noticed that the tick was engorged from its blood meal. As a result, its body was about the size of a small pea. She quickly thought about what she was going to do about this embedded tick. She decided to call the doctor's office for advice. The doctor on call said to put a hot match on it, and it should come out. Since the tick was in a hard-to-reach area of her body, she was unable to remove it herself by any method, let alone a hot match. She needed help if she was going to get that tick off her arm.

After failing to summon a friend to her home to help her, she noticed that a neighbor lady's lights were still on, so she asked her if she would help remove the tick. The woman was not comfortable attempting this, but her visiting niece volunteered to remove it. Nancy accepted the niece's help readily. Several matches were lit, one after another, and applied to the back of the tick's body, but the tick would not back out of its divot.

Nancy then asked for a pair of tweezers and requested that the two ladies not talk to her about the tick during the removal procedure since she was becoming a little panicky over the whole thing. "We laughed and joked as they attempted to pull it out. It was kind of like a little party. Though I knew that I could get sick from it, I was not really worried. I thought it was kind of a big joke," Nancy said.

When they had finally removed the tick, its body looked flattened. The ladies agreed that it did not look as engorged as it was while embedded, but no one seemed to understand the significance that this fact held for Nancy. She put it in a jar in case she would need it later. The tiny creature was walking around in the jar and looked whole, so Nancy felt reassured that no part of the tick remained in her arm.

The next day, the tick was dead in the jar. Seeing no need to keep a dead deflated tick, Nancy just threw it away. Then she examined her arm, and she noticed that it looked improved with no conspicuous inflammation. Only the tiny divot remained as evidence of this alarming incident. Just to be on the safe side, Nancy decided to check the appearance of her arm each day. What she looked for was the classic rash or bull's-eye mark indicative of Lyme disease. There was nothing remarkable about the arm, and she eventually forgot to check after a while.

Serious Symptoms Appear

By late afternoon on the 10th day, Nancy suddenly remembered that she had not checked her arm lately. When she did so, she discovered a small red bump at the site of the bite. She quickly called her doctor's office and spoke with the nurse about the tick bite and resulting red bump on her arm. The nurse told her that it could well be the beginning of Lyme disease and asked her about any systemic symptoms.

At that time, Nancy did not feel she had any symptoms to report. Despite this, the nurse made an appointment for her to come in for an exam the following day.

An hour after she concluded her phone consultation with the nurse, however, Nancy began to feel the onset of a headache, fatigue, and a sensation of mental lethargy. She decided to go to a nearby immediate care clinic. After telling her medical history to the attending physician and showing the bite site to him, she said, "I believe I have Lyme disease." She was asked if she had a rash or if she had saved the tick. She replied negatively to both questions. Since she did not have the bull's-eye rash typical of Lyme disease, the physician said that she did not have the infection.

"I felt pretty dismayed," Nancy said. Before leaving immediate care, she told the physician that the nurse at her primary doctor's office said that she could have Lyme disease and that she would be treated for that upon confirmation of the diagnosis. "The doctor left the room for a while and then came back, giving me a prescription for 200 mg [daily] of doxycycline," Nancy explained.

Nancy's drive home from the immediate care clinic was difficult. She became confused and lost her way on an otherwise familiar route. She was also shaken emotionally from the unexpected resistance she faced from the attending physician at the clinic. Drawing some comfort from the thought that she had received some antibiotics out of that argumentative encounter, she tried to put it all behind her. The next day, she called and cancelled her appointment with her primary care doctor. She thought everything was going to be just fine now. However, "as I was soon to discover, this was only the beginning of a very difficult time."

As it turned out, the prescription of doxycycline lasted two weeks. "During that time, I improved, having less fatigue, and I was feeling well enough to resume hiking.

But I still had a headache, so I went in to see my primary doctor hoping to get more medicine." Nancy went to the office armed with books from the public library about Lyme disease. She wanted to be prepared, "just in case I needed them, for I was beginning to see that the doctors were not very savvy about the disease."

Physician Resistance

Nancy's doctor listened to her explain about the tick bite and her treatment at the immediate care clinic. He then left the examining room briefly and returned with a large book on infectious diseases which included Lyme disease. He pointed out photos of the typical rash that is indicative of the infection. He also showed her the *Physician's Desk Reference* and the standard treatment for Lyme disease.

Nancy tried to direct his attention to her articles and what they said about extended and open-ended treatment, but he was not impressed. She recalled, "He told me that he would give me one more week of doxycycline, but that he wanted me to also make an appointment with an infectious disease specialist. [He] added that if I was well in one week, then I did not have Lyme disease." She was grateful for the extension of the doxycycline prescription, but she was beginning to distrust the physicians for their rigid approach to this disease.

She continued to improve during the third week of treatment, but she also began to experience strong waves of anxiety that would come and go. Confused, she wondered if these bouts of anxiety had anything to do with an earlier bee sting incident she experienced while working out in her yard. She had always been sensitive to bee stings, but usually common over-the-counter antihistamines controlled this problem.

By early June, she had taken all of her medicine and

could not understand the significance of these persisting anxiety attacks. Except for these attacks, she felt better for a short time. "I did okay for perhaps a week, but then I was sicker than ever and took to my bed." Up until then, Nancy had been working part-time at jobs arranged through a temp service, but when she required bed rest, she had to quit working altogether.

Nancy's symptoms soon began multiplying at an alarming rate. She had never before had so many symptoms plaguing her concurrently or with this degree of intensity. "Besides a severe headache, for which I was taking double doses of Ibuprofen and sleeping on two pillows to elevate my head without relief, I was very fatigued. [I] had sore throat with swollen glands, especially in front of my left ear; eye pain and dryness; pain at the juncture of the spine and head, which was especially uncomfortable; aching and shooting pains in all my limbs; and massive muscle twitches that jerked my legs." She also experienced angina-like pains, arrhythmias, stomach pain, and cognitive impairment including memory loss and dyslexia. Understandably, she also suffered from depression. "I felt very alone," she remembered.

Desperate for help, Nancy decided to return to immediate care for another evaluation. "I sat in the waiting room a long time feeling very foggy-brained and sick. Finally, I was seen by a woman doctor who gave me pretty much the same song-and-dance I had gotten before...'You do not have Lyme disease.'" This doctor also retrieved her resource books and showed Nancy the rash that precedes the disease symptoms, drawing to her attention that this rash was not present in Nancy's case. Recalling that tense moment, Nancy said, "By now I knew a few things. I told her that not everyone develops the typical rash, and [I] told her that I was very sick but had been getting well when taking doxycycline. I pleaded to have more medicine."

175

The physician cautiously suggested that she wanted to test her blood before she agreed to prescribe more antibiotics. But Nancy told her that blood work at this juncture might not provide reliable results because of her having already taken antibiotics. Still, the doctor insisted, and Nancy ultimately cooperated. It was a moment of anticipated failure for Nancy. "She [the physician] left the room in a huff, slamming the door. I am sure she did not like being instructed by one of her patients. I sat and cried. I felt so weak and desperate."

When the physician returned to the room, she told Nancy that the blood work did not show any evidence of Lyme disease. Yet she agreed to give Nancy medicine anyway. Mistakenly thinking that her previous anxiety attacks might have been an allergic reaction to doxycycline, Nancy mentioned this to the physician who then gave her a prescription for amoxicillin.

To her dismay, she did not fare well on her new prescription. "Now I was very sick. The amoxicillin did not seem to help as much as the doxycycline had. My days now consisted of doing the minimum necessary to sustain myself—taking medicine and resting in bed." She could not help but compare her present state to the person she used to be. "I had [once] been a strong, outdoors woman, hiking miles per day, hoisting heavy packs up large mountains, and now I could hardly walk around the block. I was so fatigued."

The Infectious Disease Specialist

Returning to a book she had already studied on the subject, Nancy noticed a list of Lyme disease support groups in the appendix. She called one listed in the Portland, Oregon area. Dr. Rita Stanley answered that call, and they engaged in a long conversation about Nancy's medical history. Nancy said, "She [Dr. Stanley] taught me, encouraged me, and strengthened me." It was the ray of hope that Nancy needed to continue her search for a knowledgeable physician who would employ a curative treatment protocol for her.

But first, since Nancy felt that she had not yet consulted with an infectious disease specialist, she made an appointment to see one. "The infectious disease specialist was as implacable as all the rest. He rhetorically asked me if I knew how little Lyme disease there was in Oregon. I offered him some Lyme disease literature that I had, but he didn't want it. No matter what I said, he did not want to listen. I broke down and cried."

Angered at the inflexibility of this specialist, she boldly told him that he didn't know what he was talking about. In response, he suggested doing some blood work. Nancy submitted to his idea just in case something became evident in the tests. Eight large tubes of blood were collected and tests were run.

When Nancy returned for a follow-up appointment with the specialist, he informed her, "I don't know what you have, but you don't have Lyme disease." Though not surprised at his conclusion, Nancy was infuriated and discouraged. She left the doctor with some recommendations for study on Lyme disease and never returned to his office again.

The Reluctant Physician

After consulting with Dr. Stanley again, Nancy made an appointment with a physician in a nearby city. "This appointment was not as easy as I had hoped either," Nancy said. He lectured Nancy in the now-too-familiar diagnostic guidelines for Lyme disease. She promptly broke down and cried. "I felt as if I could not take it anymore. The hardness of heart exhibited by the medical community was at least as difficult to bear as the disease itself, perhaps more so. I don't ever remember feeling so alone, rejected, and uncared for as I did during this period of time when I was seeking treatment for this disease," confessed Nancy. It was almost unfathomable to her that someone as ill as she was could not find a sympathetic, competent doctor to help her.

In spite of the doctor's initial, harsh presentation, he did ultimately prescribe doxycycline for Nancy. On the second visit to this doctor, Nancy was accompanied by Dr. Stanley as her advocate and educational intermediary during this patient-doctor meeting. The doctor listened to the suggestions and showed a willingness to run a number of critical tests and to opt for an open-ended approach in treatment.

However, the physician was quite aware of the risks he was taking in Nancy's case. He knew that physicians could place their medical licenses in jeopardy for treating Lyme disease patients with open-ended and extended antibiotic therapies. In fact, he was so reluctant and apprehensive about treating Nancy in this manner, that he turned away another Lyme patient as a result.

With every subsequent visit to this doctor's office, Nancy was subjected to the same harsh opening lecture on Lyme disease. Testing eventually supported the diagnosis, and her treatment was modified as she progressed. As a result, she continued to improve as the months wore on. She also took dietary supplements and a probiotic formula during her antibiotic treatment. In this way, she avoided an overgrowth of gastrointestinal yeast common to long-term antibiotic users. As her symptoms abated, so did her depression and emotional sensitivity to the physician's reputation-guarding lectures. She was feeling stronger again, though not without having gone through a number of symptom aggravations.

Initially, Nancy felt confident that these flare-ups would not affect her adversely. But one afternoon during her treatment period, she felt suddenly very sick, as if she was going to faint and perhaps even die. She took a Benadryl and laid down to rest. From bed she called Dr. Stanley who was able to reassure her that temporary flares were a common occurrence. She also encouraged Nancy to have her physician closely monitor her condition and to take any downturns seriously.

In addition to the local support she received, Nancy relied upon her own tested qualities of perseverance and endurance that she had cultivated as a young girl living in Minnesota. She drew strength from knowing these qualities had helped her numerous times before in ill health, and there was no reason to believe they would not serve her well now. Sometimes an illness can appear as large as a mountain, but Nancy knew with confidence that even the largest mountain could be climbed one step at a time, one axe jam at a time.

Reaching the Summit

By the summer of 1999, Nancy had improved to the point where she could perform her normal household activities again. Her illness and financial restraints necessitated relocation in October to a smaller residence—not a small feat for a Lyme patient. "When I look back on it, I do not see how I did it," she said. However, necessity is the mother of all sorts of accomplishments in life. Some things must be done, and somehow they get done. In any case, this was not the last of Nancy's accomplishments.

With the summit of good health now clearly in view, Nancy made unrelenting advancement toward it. In the process, she also experienced a spiritual conversion that helped her cope during her treatment. "Even though I was physically ill, I was filled with joy, and my heart was turned toward spiritual things. I subsequently went back to church." That fall, she attended the Multnomah Biblical

Seminary in Portland, where she completed the first year of her Master's degree work. What a climb from brain-fog to cognitive accomplishment!

One and a half years after the initial tick bite, Nancy Oace reached the summit of her recovery. Though she had forsaken mountain climbing for pursuits more important to her, she said, "I do walk every day, and [I] have done a few hikes and cross-country skis. [I am] fairly strong when I take part in these activities. For all practical purposes, I believe that my body has overcome the disease." Today, Nancy is working part-time and actively associating with her congregation, family, and friends.

Lessons Learned

As Nancy educated herself about ticks and Lyme disease, she realized that perhaps her own illness could have been minimized had she known how to remove an attached tick properly. She explained, "The appropriate way to remove a tick is to use a straight tweezers with tips that come to a rather fine point. The tweezers should be held parallel to the skin. This is very important...grasp the tick at the point where it is attached, as close to the skin as possible. Gently pull on the tick just enough to encourage it to release and wait patiently."

A very real and serious danger lies in grasping a tick by its plump body when trying to remove it with a tweezers. Nancy explained what typically happens if the tick's body is compressed in the removal process, "Its body fluids, which may include disease bacteria, will be expelled into the bloodstream increasing risk of systemic infection. This is what happened to me."

Other methods of removal, such as applying Vaseline or hot matches or anything else to the tick, may also result in the tick disgorging its body fluids and disease bacteria into the bite site. Such methods are entirely incorrect and should never be employed by anyone or suggested to anyone who has an attached tick. In Nancy's case, the tick's flattened body appearance, following removal, clearly showed that improper removal techniques emptied the tick of its contents, and this may have been the reason why she got so ill so quickly.

There are commercial tick removal devices available through some outdoor equipment stores. The tips slide around the mouthpiece of the tick next to the skin. For those who are frequently outdoors, Nancy advises carrying a plastic pill bottle or lightweight container in which to capture the biting tick. Ticks can be tested later if there is any question about infection. Lastly, "Always swab the area of the bite with alcohol or an antibacterial wipe," Nancy said.

The Prudent Pupil

There is no greater schoolmaster than experience. It instructs at great cost but teaches as no other. Nancy Oace became an unsuspecting pupil when she contracted Lyme disease in May 1998. During her illness and treatment, she gained valuable knowledge that may help anyone facing similar circumstances. She advised, "Contact the Lyme support group in [your] area by checking with the hospitals. Read up on the subject in books [in order to] judge whether you are getting good treatment and being diagnosed correctly or at all. It would be especially difficult to go through this particular disease without knowledgeable support to counteract all of the misinformation that is out there, most notably among those in the medical community."

If a person exhibits the symptoms of Lyme disease, she warns, "Do not, I repeat, do not listen to your doctor when he tells you that you don't have Lyme disease. [This disease] is supposed to be diagnosed by symptoms, and very few doctors even know what the symptoms are." Blood tests are only a part of the entire clinical picture in diagnosing Lyme disease as was seen in Nancy's case. As other pupils of the illness have learned, diagnosing Lyme disease involves a thorough clinical evaluation of symptoms, careful and meaningful testing, correct test interpretation, elimination of other possible causes, and listening—really listening—to what the patient says.

Nancy also learned there is a direct correlation between early diagnosis and treatment and the degree to which a patient recovers. It can be the difference between a cure and suffering with a chronic illness. She pleaded, "Get treatment as quickly as possible and stick with it!" It was indeed a fight for life as she expressed it, "Having this disease is like going to war." Nancy won her war, but she realized, sadly, that many of the battles could have been minimized if a less rigid approach to the diagnosis and treatment of Lyme disease was acknowledged more fully by the medical community.

A Summer Sucked Away
by Nancy Oace
July 1998

Borrelia burgdorferi,
Finely coiled worms,
Nematodes to be
Spewed from mouths
Of arthropods.

Alien mouths,
Stick-like mouths
Anesthetizing biters.

Thumbing rides
From waving weeds;
Grasping legs
From grassy stalks;
Sawing openings
In unwilling skin.

Borrelia burgdorferi,
Uninvited visitors
Pulsing through my blood;
Lodging in my cells
Multiplying.

How many did you carry,
You vile blood-sucking parasite,
When you bit me?

Swollen sucking tick
Bloated like a pea,
Leaving your legacy
Drinking on me.

I'd like to lay you down
On the hard cold concrete
And smash you to a pulp.

Disgusting dirty creature!

You stole my health;
A summer sucked away
By an alien invader.

A Year Ago I Climbed
by Nancy Oace
July 1998

A year ago
I climbed mountains.
I climbed Mt. Rainier
With forty-eight pounds
On my back.
Almost hit by rock fall,
I lived to tell it.

This year I climb nothing.

A year ago I saw friends
Three times a week, sometimes four.
We chattered up and down the trails,
Scrambled up and slid down shale.

This year there's only me.

A year ago I had big plans:
Going to take cross-country ski class.
Going to climb in Mexico;
This year though,
There's just one thing that I know:
I will be spending a lot of time in bed
And very little elsewhere go.

This year I have Lyme disease.

The wrong tick bit in May.
I was out for the day.
I was so strong!
My legs pumped up hills,
I breathed deep and full.
It felt good to use my body so.
These days it is hard
To make it past my yard.

I haven't hiked a day,
I've cancelled all my climbs,
Borne weakness, aches, and pains
With rather singular stoicism,
I'd say.
But today I cried,
Because I realized,

My body will not carry me
Up those mountains now.

If not now, when?
Don't know, don't know.

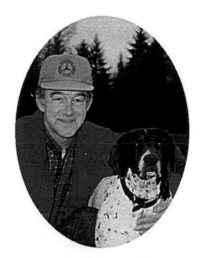

Miguel and Bo

Miguel and Super Bo Fur Hall

"Compassion is the language that even the
deaf can hear and the blind can see."
—*R. Wallen*

It was time for a lifestyle change, and that's when
Miguel first met Bo. Miguel Perez-Lizano, 49,
a technology analyst with IBM, decided it was
time to leave San Francisco after living there for 42 years.
His opportunity came in 1990, when he noticed a 40 acre
farm listed for sale in Battle Ground, Washington. It was
the perfect country residence, and with the extra acreage,
Miguel thought it was an attractive investment opportunity.

"It was a beautiful property with a creek on one side
and, in the center, a three acre, spring-fed pond stocked
with rainbow trout. My plan was to build a luxury home

overlooking the pond," Miguel said. On further inspection of the property, he also noticed a German Shorthair Pointer, the only dog remaining in the kennels on the estate. The widow, who was selling the property, cared very little for the dog she called Bo—after all, overseeing him was one of the mundane duties of the caretaker. After she fired the caretaker two years earlier, neighbors say that Bo never saw the outside of his kennel again.

Bo's papered name was Super Bo Fur Halb, and he was born on the farm Thanksgiving Day 1985. He belonged to the widow's late husband, an outdoorsman, who had taken Bo everywhere with him. On one rare traveling occasion, Bo was left behind at home. Though accustomed to riding on planes with his master, he was not invited this time. It was a decision that saved Bo's life. The plane crashed on that fateful trip, and Bo's master never returned.

Now Bo's days were spent alone in a four by twenty foot chain link kennel. From there he viewed the farm and its occasional visitors—no more car rides, no more airplane rides, no more outdoor adventures, no more companion. Occasionally, he saw the real estate agent showing people around the farm. He barked, but nobody ever stayed.

Then one day, the real estate agent showed the farm to Miguel. Bo stood on his hind legs and banged the gate of his kennel with his front paws trying to capture Miguel's attention. How could anyone who loved animals, as Miguel did, resist that kind of pleading? Miguel responded compassionately by unlatching the gate and taking Bo for a walk—a simple act that bonded them for life.

The widow originally wanted to sell Bo apart from the real estate. However, Miguel negotiated with her, and in the final settlement, she decided to throw the dog in with the deal. "So that's how I got Bo. He became my constant companion, and [he] never set foot in the kennel again," Miguel said.

Traveling Partners

During the next four years, Bo went everywhere with Miguel. It was amusing to Miguel that wherever they went, Bo always attracted the attention of the ladies. Miguel teased, "[Bo] hurt my feelings—for a long time I thought the ladies were coming up to pet him so they could talk to me. Then I found out it was really him they found attractive! One time, he managed to corner three airline stewardesses at Timberline Lodge [in Oregon]. They hardly paid any attention to me."

In May of 1994, Miguel took Bo on their first, long, road trip to Arizona where Miguel wanted to visit friends, go hiking, and do a little treasure hunting. "I like Western history and [enjoyed] researching treasure tales," he explained. As they traveled a route through northern California, Miguel stopped frequently at rest stops to walk with Bo, thinking he would need a break from the confines of the Bronco.

Everything seemed to go well until Miguel reached his friend's home in Arizona. There they were confronted with immediate trouble from the neighbor's dog. "On jumping out of the Bronco, a large dog circled around and attacked Bo. He could barely walk and required 35 stitches on his leg, so he never went on hikes with me during the trip," Miguel said.

For the rest of the trip, Bo didn't feel like doing much of anything. While Miguel went hiking, Bo rested. Miguel didn't think anything was peculiar about Bo's lethargic disposition, considering what he had just been through. However, on their route back home, before they reached Los Angeles, Bo began to act strangely. "He did not want to go back into the Bronco," Miguel recalled. Since Bo didn't tolerate heat well, Miguel simply thought that was the reason for his odd behavior. Once he coaxed Bo back into the vehicle, though, Miguel didn't give it any more thought.

A Circular Rash

The long drive home was again punctuated by frequent rest stops along the way, but eventually they made it back to their farm. "We made it home, and shortly after [that], I started to feel bad," said Miguel. It was then that he noticed a circular rash about 10 cm in diameter on the right side of his chest. Recalling this, he said, "[I] remembered a feeling of dread. I felt lousy, but not terrible. I was always the type to tough things out rather than see a doctor." He toughed it out this time, too, and the rash faded away along with Miguel's concern.

Oddly, when he noticed his own rash, he also noticed about one-fourth of a circular rash on Bo's tummy. Miguel was planning to take Bo to the veterinarian's office for an exam, but since Bo's rash disappeared quickly, and he was acting normally, he thought it was a harmless, self-limiting insect bite.

The appearances of their similar looking rashes occurred in May 1994, when Miguel was still enjoying a temporary hiatus from financial projects. "I was planning to develop this property, [and] I was planning to either start another investment management business with my friend in Seattle, continue providing technology research for institutional clients, or do something else in the investment field." Despite his ambitious intentions, the months following the appearance of his rash introduced a period of immobilization for both Bo and Miguel.

With a gradual onset, Bo and Miguel began to experience oddly similar cardiac, neurologic, and arthritic symptoms. "We had almost identical symptoms, and I never made the connection," Miguel said. Miguel's symptoms first began to appear later in 1994 with dental problems that required a root canal. Then in 1995, Miguel noticed that he was often short of breath, and that he had pain in his right shoulder.

Bo's symptoms became so painfully obvious that Miguel eventually took him to the veterinarian. Along with arthritic and muscular pain, the veterinarian noted that Bo's heart rhythm was irregular, and she diagnosed Bo's condition as a canine form of multiple sclerosis. Miguel had no reason to question this, so he accepted his companion's sad diagnosis as fact.

Ambitions on Hold

Miguel's symptoms continually worsened until, in 1996, he started experiencing frequent episodes of ventricular tachycardias of 250 or more beats per minute. "[This] resulted in more trips to the emergency room than I can remember. [Also] my memory and mental function were so impaired [that] I would get lost in my own home," Miguel said.

Physically incapacitated and virtually homebound, the economist, Miguel, regretfully could not cash in on the wildest stock market mania of the century. Instead, the booming '90s were very quiet years for Miguel. "I dropped all of these [business] pursuits. I told my friend in Seattle that I simply didn't have the energy to start new investment management firms [in Seattle and Portland]. I was not able to think well enough to develop my investment models."

For someone like Miguel—with an MBA in finance from Berkeley and a previously successful investment venture in San Francisco—this aggressive illness was a thief of life, liberty, and the pursuit of dreams. Were his business accolades simply a flash-in-the-pan display of innovative genius—short-lived and now cruelly robbed by ill health? He hoped that would not be the case. However, when comparing his former abilities and achievements to his current state of being, he could not deny that a widening chasm existed.

Working for IBM as a systems engineer and later a technology analyst, was without a doubt, mentally stimulating. His two major accounts, Stanford University and Stanford Research Institute, had a technology wish list that occupied most of his time. "IBM would assign me projects that required innovation. The project at Stanford was the great granddaddy of home computing," Miguel said. Though notably modest about his achievements, in reality, some of the hardware and software concepts that he helped create were so impressive, that in 1965, *Life Magazine* and other magazines published articles about them.

Miguel's innovative achievements also included the creation of an automated fare mechanism for the Bay Area Rapid Transit system. In this project, he helped engineer the idea of using a magnetic read/write stripe on a stiff medium. The idea was ingenious and enduring because the same automated fare machines are still in use today by that transit system.

Probably the most infamous of Miguel's business anecdotes, however, was one in which he met privately with Intel founders and innovators, Bob Noyce and Gordon Moore. During this meeting, they were discussing the potential use of the microprocessor. Puzzled, neither Noyce nor Moore could immediately think of how the microprocessor could be employed. "I remember vividly sitting there and thinking—why not make a small computer? After all, this was simply an extension of my IBM project. But I decided it was a dumb question, and these guys were really smart, so I never asked it," said Miguel with amusement.

Decades of innovations have made their debut since then, and Miguel played a modest part in that evolving technology. Then he retired from IBM, but he never rested from his private aspirations. "I was exploring [the idea of] starting a consulting venture for technology stock analysis— developing some innovative ideas I had for technical analysis of the markets using computers," he explained. That was then, but now all of those ambitions were suddenly on hold.

Symptoms Multiply

Miguel's symptoms were multiplying at a frightening pace. The year 1996 had brought on more episodes of tachycardia, shortness of breath, and a bout with pneumonia. He also experienced jaw pain, constant fatigue, a change in metabolism and appetite, chills, and heat flushes. In 1997, he noticed significant muscle fatigue in his legs. His vision was also obstructed by frequent and annoying floaters. By 1998, Miguel complained of a persistent stiff neck and joints that creaked and cracked when he moved.

Then in 1999, his knees became very painful to move, and he felt a tingling sensation in his back, neck, and scalp. There were also other symptoms that seemed mysteriously unrelated yet persisted concurrently with all the others. These included ringing in his ears, intermittent hearing loss, lethargy, a decrease in voice strength, severe sinus congestion, mucous discharge, a foul taste in his mouth, and persistent foot fungus.

Additional vision problems developed as well. Not only did he have floaters that blocked his vision, but his vision became intermittently blurred as well. He also felt an odd sensation of pressure in his eyes. Consequently, Miguel consulted with an ophthalmologist who examined him for these complaints. The physician diagnosed Miguel's condition as sixth cranial nerve palsy and optic neuritis.

The musculoskeletal impairments and the visual problems were significant enough in terms of impeding Miguel's lifestyle, but when his symptoms became neurologically involved, he became truly frightened. Ever since 1998, he had noticed that he had difficulty concentrating, but two years later, that condition developed into a much more debilitating "brain fog" along with frequent episodes of spatial disorientation, dizziness, and decreased short-term memory recall. For a man whose mind had successfully served him for many decades in a profession requiring highly analytical thinking, these symptoms were signs of an alarming invasion into the core of his very being.

By the year 2000, Miguel's symptoms numbered 29 distinct ailments, involving five different body systems. His condition had immobilized him for all practical purposes, and he seldom left the house. "Basically, I spent the whole day laying down and taking care of Bo," he said.

It wasn't that he surrendered to his illness—no, in fact, he had seen many doctors and specialists during those six years from 1994 through 2000. Like many people seeking curative treatments, Miguel trusted physicians and thought they were honest and competent professionals. He realized they were not gods, and that a reasonable amount of testing and medical theorizing accompanied this profession, and he was trying to be patient.

Still, the bottom line was that none had been able, so far, to diagnose his strange illness. "The doctors at [my HMO] focused on my cardiac problems. In the process, I was given orally inhaled steroids for breathing problems and injected steroids for arthritic problems. When these were discontinued, my symptoms exploded in severity. It was all I could do to take care of Bo and myself," Miguel remembered.

My Buddy Bo

Bo was in terrible health by spring of 2000. He could no longer walk—his muscles and joints hurt so badly. Miguel knew it was time to perform his last coup de grace toward his old friend. As he pet Bo's speckled body, his mind sped back to memories of happier days, to the beginning of their shared history—when introductions were first exchanged. There was four-year-old Bo, standing on his hind legs in that kennel, banging on the gate for release from his long confinement and neglect. It seemed like just yesterday.

Now, in the living room of the house, Miguel would free Bo again—this time, from his confinement to pain and suffering. Recalling that day, Miguel said, "I called the vet to come to the house and put him down. Bo was put down on Good Friday, 2000, in the living room—the same room where he was born. He was my buddy for 10 years." Miguel grieved deeply for his lost companion.

His still body was removed from the house for cremation. "My daughter scattered his ashes on the pasture by the pond where he loved to run." It was an appropriate place for Bo, Miguel thought. Now whenever he thinks of Bo, he visualizes him racing wildly across that pasture, legs fully extended, his liver colored ears flapping with the wind and having the time of his life!

Over the years, small anecdotes of life with Bo have recycled in Miguel's mind—many of them quite humorous. He can still recall one time when Bo was traveling with him and sitting upright in the front passenger seat of the vehicle— an onlooker saw "the passenger" from behind and mistook Bo for an unscrupulous brunette in the company of Miguel. Scandalous! In Bo's absence, such memories continue to bring laughter and comfort to Miguel's heart.

Attending to Self

After Bo's death, Miguel knew that he had to discover what was causing his own illness. He said, "I told myself that when it was time to put Bo to sleep, I would [either] find out what was wrong with me or die. The symptoms became quite exaggerated when [my HMO] took me off [the] steroids that I was on for a few months." It was apparent that the medical professionals he had consulted had not yet come to an accurate diagnosis. Miguel had been patient so far, trusting that these physicians would succeed in diagnosing his illness. However, Miguel's health had deteriorated so badly, that he *finally* realized that he had to become more involved in the search for a correct diagnosis.

He started his search on the Internet. "It took me about 30 minutes on the Internet to figure out what I had. I came across Dr. John Bleiweiss' paper, *When to Suspect Lyme Disease*. He had a patient with symptoms almost identical to mine. [Then] the significance of the rash became quite apparent." Now, sadly, he also understood what had killed Bo.

Reflecting back on where he might have come in contact with infected ticks, Miguel said, "The only places we walked in grassy or brushy areas during that trip were at interstate highway rest areas in Oregon and California. This was the most likely place of infection, and I frequently wonder how many others are being infected with this disease and other tick-borne diseases at these rest areas."

After this realization, Miguel read about the standard of treatment for Lyme disease. Leaning more toward natural methods of healing, Miguel first implemented a 6-month regimen of herbal supplements to help rebuild his immune system. He continued this from May 2000 until November, and to his great relief, he noticed that some symptoms were subsiding.

Along with this regimen, Miguel also knew that he would need the professional help of a physician to arrest the more aggressive symptoms of his widely disseminated Lyme disease. He tried to get an appointment with his primary care physician. "For about one month, I tried to get an appointment...[but] he refused to see me when he learned it was about Lyme disease. Finally, he referred me to an infectious disease specialist [in San Francisco]."

Since he could not get in to see the specialist until June, Miguel acquired some antibiotics from a private source and began a self-treating protocol. His objective was to strengthen himself to endure the long trip to San Francisco. However, eighteen hours after starting this antibiotic regimen, he experienced what appeared to be a serious Herxheimer reaction in the form of a four hour long episode of chest pain.

Miguel stopped taking the amoxicillin immediately, and when his symptoms subsided, he began taking tinidazole in its place. This antibiotic seemed to eliminate the ventricular tachycardias, and within a few weeks, his body temperature rose back up from 96.8 to 98.6. After a month on tinidazole, he replaced that antibiotic with two others, doxycycline and minocycline—one at a time, alternating these with natural remedies.

Heart Disease

After that frightening episode of chest pain, Miguel realized that the Lyme spirochetes must have infected his heart, so he made an appointment to consult with a cardiologist. At this appointment, Miguel expressed his concern about possibly having Lyme disease. The cardiologist responded compassionately, yet in a very guarded way. Miguel said, "He really helped me but asked me to leave him out of the Lyme issue."

Miguel was no stranger to cardiologists. In 1982 after a heart attack, he was diagnosed with congenital hypertrophic cardiomyopathy (HCM—enlargement and thickening of the heart muscle, existing at birth). "I was always short-winded from it. I was prohibited from playing basketball at Berkeley, although at the time, the doctors did not know exactly what was wrong with me. Even at my best physical condition, while doing track at Berkeley, I could only jog one lap before getting winded. I have always had problems with stamina, even without doing exercise," Miguel explained.

The heart attack he suffered in 1982 damaged some of his heart tissue, but after that event, he had no further heart problems of any kind. Then, in 1996, he experienced some heart arrhythmias (irregular heart rhythms); and in 1998, a blockage was identified, and an arterial stent was put in place. The rapid onset of this blockage seemed suspicious to Miguel, but he was led to believe that its formation was a predictable progression of his congenital heart disease. He did not know then what part Lyme disease could have played in this development.

As he became more knowledgeable about Lyme disease, he learned that it is well documented to cause adverse effects on the heart. Between 10-20% of Lyme disease patients develop cardiac complications. Various heart conditions may develop including: slowing down so a pacemaker is needed, fast or irregular heart beats, a swelling or enlarged heart from infection, heart related fatigue, shortness of breath, diminished exercise tolerance, dizziness or light-headedness, and chest discomfort. Heart blockages may form where the ventricles beat independently of the atrial chambers and result in decreased cardiac output. Problems arise from direct infection of the heart and/or from the effects of the disease on the innervation of the organ.

Sudden death is a grave risk among Lyme disease patients with cardiac infection. Since chest pain is not uncommon in patients with Lyme disease, it is sometimes difficult to recognize a threatening angina from intracostal pain or referred pain from the gastrointestinal tract or liver. For those who do not quickly recognize when emergency intervention is required, death may result. Not surprising then, that the autopsies of some Lyme disease patients, who have died of apparent heart failure, have shown evidence of Lyme spirochete residence in the heart.

Miguel needed no convincing of these facts. "The most serious cardiac problem I had from Lyme disease was ventricular tachycardia. I have EKG strips showing a heart rate of 300 bpm. At this speed, the heart is just quivering and blood is not being pumped. I almost lost consciousness a number of times. One month of taking tinidazole resolved this," he said.

An Inhibiting Presence

Finally, in June 2000, Miguel met with the infectious disease specialist in San Francisco. (This physician was a participating HMO healthcare provider.) After the examination, the physician reported that "in his opinion, [Miguel's symptoms] were not consistent with Lyme disease." He based his opinion heavily upon the negative results of the ELISA performed by Miguel's insurance company's contracted laboratory.

However, Miguel was puzzled why this specialist seemingly minimized the evidence of Miguel's erythema migrans (EM) rash—which the Centers for Disease Control and Prevention (CDC) consider a hallmark symptom of Lyme disease. In answer, the physician insisted that such rashes could be caused by "many, many, many diseases." Three times during this consultation, Miguel asked him to name one of these many diseases, and three times the physician neglected to answer.

Miguel was beginning to feel the inhibiting presence of his powerful insurance company. He wondered why his HMO physicians were prohibited from using outside laboratories for the ELISA and why he was being denied diagnosis and care for Lyme disease. The insurance company had Miguel locked into its system of restrictive surveillance and case definition policies. Of course, with pre-existing congenital HCM, Miguel was not in a position to easily change insurance carriers. Consequently, the only way he could get the healthcare and tests he wanted was to pay out-of-pocket, which he did on occasion.

In his continued attempts to get tests approved by his HMO, Miguel next consulted a neurologist. "He tried to help me by ordering the Western blot IgG and IgM tests and bypassing [the] ELISA." The neurologist understood that ELISAs are not as reliable for indicating widely disseminated Lyme disease as are Western blot tests, so he was willing to accommodate Miguel's request for these assays. Guarded this time, Miguel later asked the nurse to read the physician's orders from her notes. She did, and all seemed consistent with what Miguel and the doctor had discussed. Relieved that he would finally have more comprehensive tests performed, he went to the lab to have blood drawn.

However, a problem arose shortly thereafter. "When I went to have [my] blood drawn, this doctor's orders were apparently blocked. I could have the [HMO's] Western blot tests [performed] *only if* the ELISA was positive. The ELISA, of course, was once again negative," Miguel explained.

Fortunately, Miguel's doctor cooperated in allowing Miguel to pay out-of-pocket for a Western blot IgG test through a laboratory unaffiliated with Miguel's HMO. When the results came back from that laboratory, it showed the presence of four bands of positive intensity and one band of equivocal (uncertain) intensity. "The CDC surveillance criteria require five bands of positive intensity to meet the case definition," Miguel explained.

Surveillance data is for reporting purposes only, and the CDC stresses that. While the FDA warns about the potential for misuse of these test results in making a diagnosis, the use of these criteria have also been embraced as a serodiagnostic standard. In addition, in trials done for the Lyme vaccine study, only 22% of proven Lyme cases were able to meet the five band IgG criteria, so Miguel was not willing to dismiss Lyme disease as the cause of his illness just because his test results fell marginally short by one band out of the CDC's five band criteria.

The neurologist, who examined the IgG test results, agreed with Miguel and refused to rule out Lyme disease. "The neurologist who challenged the non-specific negative ELISA result with the IgG results was forced to defer to the infectious disease clinician—the same infectious disease clinician who [earlier] denied my diagnosis." It was unbelievable! Miguel was once again face-to-face with his previous opponent on this health issue.

The infectious disease clinician examined the Western blot IgG test results and concluded that it was not significant in that the results did not increase the probability that Miguel had "active, chronic Lyme disease in any organ system." His comment was supposedly supported by the second negative ELISA performed by the HMO's contracted laboratory. The doctor only considered the dominant two-tier testing schema (ELISA followed by Western blotting), even though this approach has been shown by others to miss a significant number of cases. The fact that a Western blot IgG test is generally more specific than the ELISA, did not seem to have any bearing on the stand taken by the infectious disease specialist.

Frustrated, Miguel said, "This denial was in contradiction to the recommendation by the National Institute of Health—that the most appropriate serologic test for prior infection with Borrelia burgdorferi, the spirochete that causes Lyme disease, is the IgG Western blot assay." The crux of the matter was the lack of a positive ELISA, which is considered essential in the two-tiered testing approach. Miguel filed complaints and also paid out-of-pocket to have an additional Western blot test—IgM—run.

The results of that test were blatantly ignored by his HMO physician, who considered this a marker of early disease only, even though the test results exceeded CDC surveillance criteria in terms of the number of positive specific bands required for case definition. As for the former Western blot IgG test results—they were mysteriously lost by the HMO's physician. Miguel had kept his patient copy and wrote letters of appeal but to no avail.

"There appears to be a strong bias against diagnosis for Lyme disease in this [HMO] institution," Miguel said. The reason?—Miguel suspected it was the high cost of treatment.

Lyme Disease Treatment

In late 2001, Miguel terminated his 27 year membership with his HMO because its physicians refused to diagnose his illness as Lyme disease. The lack of compassion shown him by this organization and its physicians would have cost him his life had he continued under their "care." His membership termination with the HMO did not leave Miguel uninsured, however. Fortunately, Miguel's wife, a pre-school, special education teacher, carried their secondary insurance through a preferred provider organization (PPO). This organization accepted Miguel's pre-existing condition and covered nearly all his expenses. Most importantly—he was allowed to choose his own healthcare provider.

Consequently, in February 2002, Miguel consulted with a doctor in San Francisco who treated Lyme disease patients. This physician listened to Miguel relate his history, examined him, and studied over the previous copies of earlier Western blot tests. After a full clinical evaluation, the physician reordered the same Western blot tests to see how they had evolved.

Not surprisingly, by this time, the results of the Western blot IgG test were CDC positive on five bands, and seven bands showed positive on the IgM test. Additional test results indicated that Miguel had no co-infections associated with his Lyme disease.

Treatment was started immediately, and Miguel showed improvement on a treatment protocol involving the use of various antibiotics. His treatment began with a prescription of Suprax and Biaxin, and later Suprax with Zithromax, which worked very well for Miguel, eliminating his vertigo.

In March and April of 2003, Miguel's doctor ordered some extensive cardiac tests to examine the health of Miguel's heart, since many of his other symptoms had completely subsided. The cardiac test results showed that his heart was functioning properly. Since he was feeling so well, and all tests seemed to indicate a restoration of health, the doctor discontinued Miguel's treatment in June of 2003.

However, later that month troubling heart symptoms reappeared. Miguel's heart experienced constant atrial fluttering and fibrillation. Returning to the doctor immediately, Miguel resumed his antibiotic therapy. After taking a combination of antibiotics that did not seem effective, the doctor ordered another change in the regimen. In October, the doctor prescribed Omnicef and Zithromax, which Miguel took for four months. This proved very effective for restoring proper brain function, but his heart symptoms persisted.

Then in September 2004, Miguel's doctor prescribed a month's dose of tinidazole and Zithromax to treat his heart symptoms. "[It's] difficult to say if it was effective," Miguel said. Despite the fact that he was unsure of his true state of cardiac health, he seemed confident enough to try going off his therapy again October 1, 2004.

Though some experimentation had been applied in Miguel's case, his greatest improvements still resulted from well established antibiotics. Tests showed that Miguel's heart function improved when he was on a continued course of antibiotics. Conversely, when his antibiotic therapy was interrupted or discontinued, his life-threatening heart symptoms reappeared.

Miguel's treatment has been an open-ended one due to the persisting relapses involving potentially serious heart symptoms. Despite this, there is evidence of improvement. Miguel has had no ventricular tachycardia for a while, and other earlier symptoms have much improved or been 100% resolved.

"Virtually all of my symptoms have disappeared except for heart problems. My right shoulder still gives me some problems, since I was [originally] bitten in the right chest area, [and later received] two rounds of steroid injections in that shoulder. Large stressors will [also] trigger some symptoms, including the heart symptoms I am experiencing."

Having conquered most of his symptoms, Miguel's fight for life is now centered primarily on his heart. He has not ruled out the possibility that a future cardiac procedure may be necessary, but he's grateful for the health he has regained. Thinking back on how far he has come in his fight against Lyme disease, he said, "At my worst, I was probably functioning [at] about 25%. Now I am about 70%, if I am careful."

The Idea Guy

Miguel, who is still called the "Idea Guy" by some in the technology and financial worlds, has redirected his innovative energies towards healing. He knows, too well, how cruelly Lyme disease can rob one of a healthful mind, heart, and soul.

Yet at the pinnacle of his physical weakness, his mind came to his rescue. Though challenged, he did his own research on the Internet and proposed the proper tests to evaluate the cause of his afflictions. He found knowledgeable help through a support group and located a compassionate physician who would treat him. He also paid out-of-pocket for tests and healthcare that should have been offered and paid for by an insurance company he had been associated with for 27 years.

Instead of receiving full support from that trusted institution, it was Miguel's self advocacy, determination, and courage that led to his getting the help he so desperately needed. He has reclaimed the greater portion of his good health, except for his heart. Of its value, Miguel quotes from *The Little Prince* by Antoine de Saint Exupery, "It is only with the heart that one can see rightly; what is essential is invisible to the eye."

Miguel Perez-Lizano, the "Idea Guy," sees perfectly with his figurative heart. His hardships have not changed the compassionate man he has always been—not even the loss of Bo, the foregoing of a career, or the neglect he suffered at the hands of a formerly trusted healthcare system could do that.

No—Miguel is even more compassionate and now wiser for his experience. "My unquestioned confidence in medical professionals has been totally shattered. Having to learn about Lyme disease in order to survive has made me aware how limited doctors are in their knowledge base. Go to a competent Lyme disease specialist [and] stay away from any medical specialists of any kind who will not acknowledge a Lyme disease diagnosis or who trivialize the severity of the disease," Miguel advised.

Miguel believes that limited knowledge within the medical community is one significant challenge Lyme patients face. However, the other weakness in the healthcare system, as Miguel sees it, is far more incriminating. "[My experience] has made me aware of corruption in medicine. An HMO like [my former one] does not like to diagnose and treat expensive, chronic conditions [like] Lyme disease.

Therefore, their solution is to avoid diagnosis. Their guidelines discourage diagnosis to minimize costs and maximize profits."

Miguel's six year battle with his HMO over a diagnosis for Lyme disease has strongly molded his advice to others. "If [a Lyme patient] is with an HMO, change plans if possible. Select a preferred provider organization (PPO) plan that allows the patient to choose his own specialists." Being free to personally choose a knowledgeable and competent physician is a critical freedom.

Despite the various roadblocks to diagnosis and treatment, Miguel encourages others now seeking Lyme disease treatment, not to give up. "I have learned that one really can be healed from a devastating bout of Lyme disease, and there are many people who are willing to help. Seek help from a local or regional support group. This help is critical. Lyme disease victims have to learn to be proactive and not rely on doctors for everything."

Miguel has achieved his own measure of recovery by following this advice. The truths he has learned through his experience, he gladly shares. The gravest truth is—Lyme disease can be a contributing cause of heart disease and death. To this truth, the experiences of Miguel and his buddy, Bo, testify.

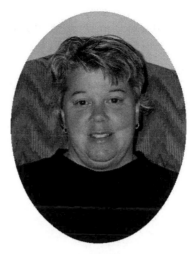

Lynda

Picture Perfect

"The best part of beauty is that which
no picture can express."
—*Frances Bacon*

Perhaps it is true that the most beautiful part of a person can never be captured on film. Outdoors woman and commercial photographer, Lynda McDonnell, 36, of Dover, Ohio, spent countless, pleasurable hours trying to capture the essence of beauty in the world around her. Yet it was only during her personal fight against Lyme disease that she discovered a beauty that could not be captured on her camera—the beauty of character jeweled with qualities reserved for times of absolute necessity.

Those times arrived when Lynda was thirty-something, and the agility of youth seemed like a distant memory. "I had always been an active kid. I was always outside playing, climbing trees, [playing] basketball, tag—whatever it was—I was busy," remembered Lynda. It was with that same kind of energy and enthusiasm that she also competed in high school tennis, basketball, and volleyball.

After high school, Lynda attended the Art Institute of Commercial Photography in Pittsburgh, Pennsylvania, where she graduated with honors in 1988. She returned to Dover, Ohio, to work in the field of photography, and there she married her husband, Bruce, the following year. As newlyweds, they had dreams of sharing many happy years together and raising a family in a home of their own.

They made their residence just outside the city limits on four acres of wooded pasture land. Three of the four acres were in pasture and brush, suitable for horses to graze. A slow moving creek meandered through the grassy pasture, providing plenty of water for their horses and a variety of mature trees including oaks, maples, poplars, cottonwoods, and some fruit trees. Groundhogs, possum, rabbits, raccoons, and snakes all found the McDonnell's property to be an inviting habitat.

However, so did the white-tailed deer and white-footed mice which posed a much greater health risk than anyone realized. At the time, Lynda knew of no one nearby who had ever contracted Lyme disease. She had heard of several cases of the disease reported within a radius of 15 miles from her home, but she did not consider herself at risk—not on her own property.

Lynda loved working outdoors in her yard and spent many hours out there. "Yes, [I enjoyed] mowing the lawn and working in mulch beds." After their son was born in 1993, she also spent time outdoors playing ball with him. She was a very active woman and loved to occupy herself outside as often as she could. "I have dogs and horses, and we are outside a lot."

Inside her home, Lynda had a number of remodeling projects that she was in the midst of completing. She enjoyed her home and felt a great deal of satisfaction in her roles as homemaker, wife, mother, gardener, and photographer. Her life was nearly picture perfect, and for the next few years, it remained just that.

In 1995, Lynda left the field of photography, and she worked as a real estate agent for four years. It was a hectic, fast-paced occupation that required clear thinking and a pleasant, business persona, assets which Lynda possessed. Her job was stimulating and financially rewarding, but it was also stressful.

To offset that stress, Lynda worked out at the local YMCA gym after dinner each evening. She also maintained a routine of walking and running, something she used to enjoy in the years following high school when she could run a seven minute mile. Now, a few years later, she found it not only enjoyable but therapeutic as well. Occasionally, she even participated in a few weekend road races. "I have always wanted to train and be able to run a marathon, and believe it or not, I still keep that in the back of my mind!"

Something's Wrong

"I was still running and walking [in 1997] when [symptoms] started [appearing]," she said. That year Lynda began feeling very odd symptoms, and she did not know their cause. "At first I was just [feeling] dopey, and that was extremely unusual. I tripped or fell up steps, stumbled, and my hands did not grip things right." She had not made the correlation between her clumsiness and a progressive disease, so she simply endured her bumbling awkwardness one day at a time.

In 1999, Lynda decided to forsake the hectic and encompassing world of real estate in exchange for more time with family and friends. She also wanted to return to photography, her first love. She lost no time in coupling photography with some fishing trips to Canada and hiking expeditions at the Cook Forest in Clarion, Pennsylvania. The trails, once so easy to traverse, now seemed to be obstacle courses. "I basically stumbled up and down those trails, but in 2000, [I] went prepared with Advil and took long hikes. [I] came back exhausted, but it was great!"

Her tenacity to enjoy the outdoors was suddenly met with an even greater challenge, extreme fatigue. "I was so tired—I mean really tired—like you just can't even move." Bruce said to her, "You look like your strings are cut." That's just how she felt, too. Her arms hurt so badly with joint pain that she could not even pick up her camera or steady it to take a photo. "All I did was sit in my chair and just hope I would feel better soon," Lynda said.

However, over the next few months, she did not improve. By the fall of 2000, her episodes of clumsiness had become so frequent and obvious that her family knew something was terribly wrong. In addition to her muscular impairments, Lynda began to feel strong pains in her lower back.

"My life really changed in January 2001, the morning I woke up and could barely get out of bed, let alone down the steps. Every joint in my body hurt, including my fingers along with a stiff neck and exhaustion!" One week previous to this, Lynda had broken out in a rash, but she thought at the time, that she had contracted fifth disease from her son and that it would soon pass. However, it didn't pass, and her life was never the same after that.

Initially, Lynda complained of joint pain, fatigue, and general malaise. As time passed, though, the list of symptoms grew to include: stiffness, shooting pains throughout her body, twitching of muscles that included her eyelids, blurred vision with floaters, stuttering, forgetfulness, word searching, feeling lost, clumsiness, numbness in her hands, restless legs, tooth pain, fevers, and nausea. Every day presented a different mix of these symptoms, and every day she felt miserably sick.

An Astute Chiropractor

Throughout the year of 2001, Lynda sought the help of many physicians. "I went from doctor to doctor and [submitted] to test after test trying to find the answer for my pain." No definitive diagnosis could be deduced despite a very extensive medical effort and the money spent by Lynda for that help.

In January of 2002, she consulted with an arthritis specialist. "He seemed baffled and tried different anti-inflammatory drugs which did not seem to help." Lynda said. Now more than ever, she disliked taking analgesic drugs. "First off, I don't feel good on those, and secondly, they have their own set of side effects." In frustration, she decided to take only Advil three times a day for pain.

Most of the diagnoses offered to Lynda by these various doctors addressed her arthritic symptoms. One doctor said she had rheumatoid arthritis, and another said she had osteoarthritis. While these seemed like credible explanations for her achy and painful joints, these explanations certainly did not address the other concurrently presenting symptoms, such as the dysfunction of her large motor skills. It was obvious to Lynda that something was being overlooked by the physicians she had seen so far.

During this time, Lynda had also been consulting with her family chiropractor. "He was very stumped by my symptoms," Lynda said. However, one day when she was in his examining room, he happened to mention that he knew another woman who had similar symptoms, and she had been diagnosed with Lyme disease. He recommended that Lynda ask one of her treating physicians about ordering a Western blot test for Lyme disease. Lynda questioned him, "But I've never had a tick on me or a rash!" Still, he encouraged her to at least inquire.

On her next visit to her physician, she asked him about the possibility that Lyme disease might be the cause of her illness. The doctor asked Lynda if she had ever had a bull's-eye rash, and she replied that she had not noticed any rash. He replied, "Then you do not have Lyme disease!"

Lynda returned to her chiropractor in January 2003 and told him that her physician did not believe she had Lyme disease because she did not observe a bull's-eye rash. The astute chiropractor understood that many Lyme disease patients did not present with a rash or might not even notice one. He explained to her that the presence or absence of a rash was only one aspect a discerning physician would consider in evaluating a patient for the disease. For this reason, he strongly encouraged her to find a doctor who would run a Western blot test for Lyme disease.

After suffering for so long and digressing in health with time, Lynda said, "At this point, I was willing to try anything as my symptoms had gone into a neurological stage, and I was scared." Her chiropractor gave her the names of two doctors he had heard about through some of his patients. Lynda then went home with the intention of researching both doctors on the Internet.

Pennsylvania Physician

Before contacting the physicians, Lynda decided to educate herself about Lyme disease. "So that night, I went on the Internet to learn about Lyme disease and its symptoms. As I pulled up the symptoms, I was just blown away by the [many] similarities. I just sat there and cried. I felt like I finally had my answer," she said. After printing off a list of symptoms, she highlighted those that she, too, had experienced. Armed with this motivating information, she was ready to make an appointment with one of the doctors recommended to her earlier.

The physician she chose to visit practiced in Pennsylvania and agreed to see her on April 23, 2003. She was willing to wait for the appointment and drive the distance because she hoped he might be the physician that would finally help her. When the day arrived, Lynda's husband accompanied her as an advocate—a second voice and another pair of ears—so that nothing would be overlooked in the process of relating her medical history to the new doctor.

After sharing her medical history with the doctor, he ordered a blood draw, and a blood sample was sent to the lab for a Western blot test for Lyme disease. After considering Lynda's case history and performing an exacting clinical evaluation, the doctor felt her presenting symptoms warranted an initial prescription of amoxicillin while they waited for the results of the test to come back. At that time, her treatment regimen would be reassessed.

Diagnosis and Treatment

On May 12, 2003, Lynda received the long-awaited call from her physician that the Western blot test results provided positive indicators for Lyme disease. At last, she knew what was causing her debilitating illness. Lynda felt relief, but she also knew that this was just the beginning. Realistically, she had a long haul ahead of her to recovery, if she could even reach it.

She believed that long-term, open-ended antibiotic therapy was necessary if she wanted to regain her health. "Believe me, I was so scared [of my symptoms] that I took the antibiotics. The first month [on treatment], I made some progress [and] after that just little bits at a time. I was on high [doses] of oral antibiotics until September 2003," she said. At that time, the doctor recommended a change to IV therapy for a period of 10 weeks. Lynda agreed to this and was started on the antibiotic, Rocephin.

Unfortunately, she could not tolerate the drug, so it was replaced with another antibiotic, Zithromax. "That was better, but a long haul," Lynda said. "I do feel that the IV therapy helped [me], but I am not symptom-free yet." In June 2004, Lynda's doctor started her on a new daily regimen of two different oral antibiotics, Biaxin and clindamycin. Then every 30 days, she saw her physician so that he could monitor her treatment progress.

In addition to her medication, Lynda modified her diet to include natural juices and herbal teas. She also took acidophilus daily to counteract any possible yeast infections that could occur with strong antibiotic use. From experience, she learned that ingesting certain foods seemed to worsen her symptoms. "Since the end of June [2003]—no sugar, breads, pasta, or other starches. This seems to be working—I feel a little better," Lynda explained.

Beating my Drums

As a result of antibiotic treatment, proper rest, and positive changes in lifestyle and diet, Lynda regained about 75% of her former good health. "I still have symptoms—I feel like a yo-yo sometimes. There are days that if I did have a job, I would not be able to go to work."

Lynda is now a stay-at-home mom, who is seemingly rarely at home. Between attending her son's school events and enrolling in adult education classes, she finds herself frequently exhausted. However, she admits, "The best thing I have going for me is a very supportive husband and son, who have been right at my side through this whole ordeal along with my mother, sister, and some super friends!"

A loving team of advocates certainly aided Lynda in achieving the progress she now enjoys. However, not to be overlooked was Lynda's self education efforts—her own inquisitive mind that searched for knowledgeable answers to a very complex disease. She credits her former competitive sports personality for her inner drive. "Because of my love for sports, there is that feeling of not being defeated, and that is how I look at this thing with Lyme disease. I just can't let it defeat me or my family. I will not own this disease!"

Though formerly a very private person, Lynda now sees it as her responsibility to speak out and help increase public awareness of her illness. "[I] decided that to tackle this stuff, I had to talk about it. After all, that's how I finally figured out what I had. If it hadn't been for a gal in our area talking to my chiropractor about her symptoms and Lyme disease, I might still be searching!"

To that end, she started a support group in the fall of 2003. She also has been offering information to the public about tick-borne diseases. Her mission has seen early success as Lynda readily admits. "One year later, it's working!" Referring to her efforts as "beating my drums," she focuses on educating others including medical professionals. "Hopefully, fewer people will suffer and be able to get help sooner and in their own community," she said.

Becoming your own advocate and doing your own research is of utmost importance in battling an undiagnosed illness, Lynda explained. "The first hurdle is figuring out what you have. The Internet became my friend for information. Always remember that you have to be your own advocate and ask the questions. If you don't like what you're hearing, ask some more."

Lynda's experience taught her that a patient benefits greatly if the physician truly listens to the patient. "Find a doctor you feel comfortable with and [who] does not have an ego." Time and again, professional arrogance leads to the wrong diagnosis and the wrong treatment—sometimes wasting years of precious time. Conversely, the most astute and successful doctors are those who maintain a measure of humility and who listen to the patient, especially when confronted with a disease such as Lyme disease that has such complex presentations.

Improving the System

After experiencing the costs of misinformation and limited knowledge, Lynda is more determined than ever to improve the system through education. Looking back at her own case history, she now recognizes the professional opinions that cost her valuable treatment time. "I would have been treated a year sooner if my arthritis doctor had listened better and been more informed. I trusted him and his answer, 'You do not have Lyme disease.' Now I wish I had known then all that I know now."

The absence of an erythema migrans (EM) rash is one of those factors that frequently confuses professional evaluation and ultimately postpones proper treatment. When Lynda's doctor told her "no rash, no Lyme disease," and when he dismissed her request for a Western blot test, Lynda felt he failed to listen to her as a patient. She now understands that he had limited knowledge of the disease. This was a major setback to her as a patient. "It took me another twelve months to revisit the thought [of Lyme disease]. [Meanwhile], it was attacking me neurologically, and that was scary!"

Informed health care professionals, who specialize in treating arthritis, are in a position to often be first to recognize Lyme disease symptoms. Why? "[They] are the first [physicians] you go to when you have severe joint pain," Lynda explained. Educating these specialists that migrating arthritic-like pain can be caused by Lyme disease may increase the frequency of correct, relatively early, diagnosis and treatment. This may, in turn, aid in arresting Lyme disease progression so that chronic debilitating illness may be avoided.

Healthcare Coalition

In addition to the support group that Lynda founded, another nonprofit organization called Community Healthcare Coalition of Stark County, Ohio, also became involved in the campaign to increase public awareness of Lyme disease. This outcome was expedited by Lynda's husband, Bruce, who approached the organization in search of information that might help Lynda after she was diagnosed in May 2003.

Recalling what happened, Bruce said, "I contacted the coalition to find out what they knew about Lyme, as they were continuously educating the public about various health issues. They had no knowledge of Lyme at that time." However, after learning that there was an urgent need to educate the medical community and the public in general, the organization quickly reacted. Bruce added, "[Since then], they have had two [educational] seminars for doctors and others focusing on Lyme disease."

Lynda was absolutely delighted to have this additional professional support. "My feeling is that we really need to educate the doctors," Lynda said. She has learned, at great cost to herself, that both patient and physician need to be well informed about tick-borne diseases. If patients are to be diagnosed early and treated properly, accurate medical information must be easily accessible. She feels that the Community Healthcare Coalition is a great step forward in that direction.

Refocus

For Lynda McDonnell, the years following her first symptoms in 1997, dramatically changed her life. Before that time, her focus was all about her family and her love for the outdoors and for capturing its beauty on film. Admittedly, her life was contented and private. It was almost picture perfect.

Today, when she looks through the lens at her own life, she has to refocus. All that she knew before had somehow become blurred. Now she sees herself differently—a woman made more frail by disease, more matured by pain. However, she also sees the supportive network of loved ones who have helped her carry her burdens and have acted as her advocates when she felt all her strings were cut.

What she could not capture on camera was the spirit with which she fought her illness. Her husband said, "Lynda has been what I would call valiant in fighting this disease. Throughout this long ordeal, she has been focused on beating it and looking ahead to life as it used to be. She has had moments or days of being down, but overall, she has maintained a great outlook. I have been very proud of her enthusiasm for life even when she had a lot of pain and fatigue."

Clearly, this kind of unfilmed beauty increases upon examination. Quiet heroism in the face of pain, hope despite dire odds, and determination that sees no limits—these are some of the enduring qualities that Lynda discovered in her personal battle against Lyme disease. Today, as Lynda's health returns to her so do her passions. She will return to an old love, her husband said. "Now that she has made some progress, she is planning to resume her photography."

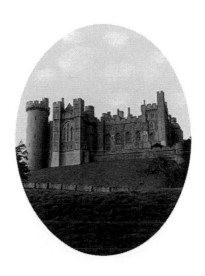

Camelot Remembered

"Those that can, do; those that can't,
cheer for those that can."
—*An Irish father*

S he comes to the ocean as often as she can. "It is a place that, for me, elicits a cascade of wonderful emotions peace, tranquility, renewal, and a sense of well being," said *Michelle O'Leary* in an undertone as she fixed her brown eyes upon the distant, tumbling waves. The white, sandy beaches of East Hampton, New York, are a spiritual refuge for her. It is her "happy place" and a place of meditation. "Everyone has such a place, I believe, where they can escape to either physically or mentally—where they can find their inner peace."

Once a month since July 2001, Michelle has sojourned to this place on her return from medical treatment for a chronic, neurologic form of Lyme disease. "I've had Lyme disease since at least 1991, perhaps even longer. It has had an impact, both positively and negatively on me, my marriage, and my family for many years," she said as she reflected upon those life changing years.

Battling a chronic condition, Michelle finds deep solace in the imagery of the ocean and its beaches. "I can be here in an instant in my mind," she whispered as a breeze of salty sea air gave spirit to her long, brown hair. The cold water lapped across the sand toward her bare feet, and almost effortlessly, the imprint of her prior steps vanished. *That's how quickly one's happy past can be erased,* she thought. She contemplated the reversal of her own personal circumstances, and she remembered happier times—in her own private Camelot—gone but not forgotten.

Early Camelot

Before her illness, she enjoyed a life that was nearly as congenial and predictable as the legendary Camelot itself. Born and educated in an affluent town in Rhode Island, Michelle was the second of three children raised in her strict, Irish Catholic family. Outnumbered by boys, both at home and in her neighborhood, she was quickly transformed into an exuberant tomboy.

In school, Michelle was involved in most of the school sports. "I was on the junior and senior varsity teams in basketball, volleyball, softball, and tennis. While other girls were primping themselves and shaking their pom-poms, I was in the training room getting my ankle taped for the upcoming basketball game." Proud of her abilities, her father told her that "those that can, do; those that can't, cheer for those that can." Every person had a role to play on game night, but Michelle later realized that this philosophy applied to a lot more than sports.

Besides being athletic, Michelle was also very talented at nurturing others. As the proverbial middle child, she became the peacemaker in the family, working hard at everything she did and trying to please everyone in the process. Her caregiving personality was well established at the age of three when she first demonstrated a keen interest in nursing. She loved to practice her medical skills on her younger brother, so it was not uncommon for her parents to find him all bandaged up by the resident nurse. Her aspirations to be a nurse continued to grow, and in almost a blink of an eye, the time arrived when she enrolled in the nursing program at the University of Rhode Island. After earning a baccalaureate of science in nursing, she took her boards in Boston and began her career as a staff nurse on a medical/surgical floor at New England Deaconess Hospital.

The unit she worked on was the inpatient arm for patients being treated at the Joslin Diabetes Center. There she began to educate patients and their families about diabetes and how to properly manage it. "I loved the teaching aspect of nursing, particularly in the field of diabetes, and I began to accumulate the years of diabetes education experience that allowed me to finally obtain my certification as a Diabetes Educator (CDE)," she said.

At twenty-eight years of age, Michelle was enjoying a successful and satisfying career in nursing; however, her parents thought that perhaps this success came at the cost of other personal pursuits, such as dating and marriage. Her mother asked her, "What benefit is there in being certified as a Diabetes Educator?" Michelle jokingly answered, "Well, it allows me to put three more letters after my name." Smiling, her mother asked, "Don't you think you should be working harder on putting three important letters before your name—like M-R-S?"

An Irish Romance

The truth of the matter was that Michelle had not yet met the right guy. That is, not until one day shortly after her conversation with her mother when she was at the health club. There she met *Kevin O'Leary*, a handsome, athletic Irishman who worked for an insurance company. In their introductory conversation, they were amused to learn that they actually lived across the street from each other. They both thought it was odd that, living in such close proximity, they had never met or even seen one another until now.

At their chance meeting, they learned that they shared an Irish ancestry and mutual interests. A definite chemistry existed between them, and a dating relationship quickly ensued. For Michelle, love was a fast fall, but not for Kevin, who had an academic agenda that took precedence for a while. He had just been accepted to Boston University School of Law, and it was such a prestigious opportunity for him that love and marriage had to take a back seat.

Although more serious commitments had to wait, their dating schedule was a busy one. They enjoyed Boston to the full, attending hockey, basketball, and football games at Boston College. Over the next couple of years, their relationship developed slowly and progressively toward a meaningful commitment.

Happily Ever-Aftering

While many fairy tales end at the altar with the proverbial "happily ever-after," Michelle's story diverted from the traditional and actually took on dramatic momentum the year she married. As for happily ever-aftering—that part of her Camelot story was yet to unfold.

For the present time, Michelle had every reason to be happy. She was in love with prospects of marriage in view. She had a wonderful job, and she was the picture of good health. However, in April 1990, Michelle experienced something very unusual. "I began having very painful, electricity-type pain starting in the middle of my back and moving across my wing bone and out to my shoulder. Sometimes the area was buzzing," she explained. She had never been ill like this before, and frankly, this condition was very bizarre.

The symptoms continued for one month before she consulted a neurologist who worked at the hospital with her. He thought perhaps she suffered from a pinched nerve, and so he ordered a magnetic resonance imaging (MRI) of her cervical spine. The results of the MRI showed nothing abnormal, so Michelle toughed it out. After about three months, the pain and buzzing went away. Even though the cause remained unknown, she was very happy that it had passed and that she could resume her work and social life.

Shortly after this incident and toward the end of Kevin's senior year in law school, he proposed to Michelle. She was so excited that she immediately told her parents the good news. "As you might imagine, my parents were ecstatic. Their daughter was [going] to marry an Irish Catholic lawyer!" They shared her joy and beamed with pride. After all, Michelle was successful in her career, financially stable, healthy, and beautiful. It seemed as if everything in her life was transpiring without a hitch.

Their wedding day finally arrived, and it took place in the fall of 1990 in Newport, Rhode Island, in the same Catholic church where, 37 years earlier, John Kennedy and Jacqueline L. Bouvier were married. The event could not have seemed more regal or the day more glorious. No expense was spared as the couple hosted an elegant reception at one of the most beautiful mansions along Ocean Drive in Newport. Every detail about their special day was romantic and picturesque. Immediately following their reception, they went happily ever-aftering to their honeymoon destination—the paradise island of Maui.

When they returned from their honeymoon, Kevin and Michelle settled into their Boston apartment and quickly established a busy routine. Kevin had just started his job as an associate lawyer in one of the two biggest law firms in Boston, and Michelle was working at Beth Israel Hospital as a Certified Diabetes Educator and researcher. Her job was challenging and exhilarating. "We were doing some cutting edge research in the field of diabetes, and working at a Harvard teaching hospital afforded me opportunities to expand my knowledge further," she said.

In their personal lives, Michelle and Kevin were eager to start a family. However, after six months, they suspected an infertility problem, and so Michelle consulted with a fertility specialist. He prescribed a two week course of doxycycline in the event that she had some ongoing bacterial infection that was preventing conception. Five days into the treatment, Michelle noticed four or five ringworm-like rashes on the back of her neck. They were about the size of a nickel, but they neither itched nor caused any pain, so she didn't bother to see a doctor. Eventually, the rashes disappeared, and Michelle gave no further thought about what might have caused them. She certainly did not suspect Lyme disease for a moment.

A Cloud over Camelot

In early February 1991, Michelle, Kevin, and six of their friends went on one of their annual skiing trips, this time near Taos, New Mexico. They rented a chalet, and for the first three days, they enjoyed the powdery ski slopes and comradery. However, on the fourth morning, Michelle woke up with an excruciating headache. Every movement made her head pound with pain, and she could barely tolerate any light. Within two hours, the pounding sensation spread down her neck and spine. Her neck felt stiff, and she became feverish.

Noticeably sick with a fever of 102 degrees and nausea, she asked Kevin to take her to the walk-in clinic in Santa Fe for evaluation. "The doctor said I probably had altitude sickness," recalled Michelle. She was discharged with instructions to drink plenty of liquids, take Motrin for the pain and fever, and rest. Although their trip ended on a disappointing note, her illness resolved on its own over the next three weeks. Again, Michelle did not know what caused this sudden onset of painful symptoms, but she hoped that was the end of it.

Two months after their Taos skiing trip, Michelle became involved in a minor car accident caused by another driver. Her car spun into an intersection, and in the process, she hit her head against the driver's side window. Fortunately, she did not lose consciousness, and she didn't experience any headaches during the remainder of that day.

Four days later, however, her entire right side became numb from the neck down. Thinking that perhaps she had injured her spinal cord in the car accident, she went to see a neurologist. The neurologist ordered a computed axial tomography (CAT) scan—a diagnostic imaging procedure— but it did not reveal any injury to her spine. Puzzled over the cause of her numbness, the neurologist conducted a thorough clinical evaluation of Michelle and discussed her medical history, including the buzzing and burning in her back that occurred in April 1990 and the illness she had experienced in Taos in February 1991.

After taking Michelle's history into account, the neurologist suspected that perhaps something systemic was going on, and she suggested that Michelle undergo a lumbar puncture. "I was petrified! My husband came with me and held my hand through the whole procedure," she recalled.

Four hours later, the results came back—there were 11 white blood cells in her spinal fluid sample—evidence, possibly, of a case of viral meningitis in the latter stages of resolving. With this information, she was sent home to rest and to observe if the right-sided numbness resolved within the next week. If not, Michelle was advised to call the doctor for another examination.

Multiple Sclerosis

Less than a week transpired since the lumbar puncture before another serious medical symptom surfaced. "I now had a decrease in my hearing on the right side. Sounds echoed, and high pitched noises were unbearable," she said. Michelle immediately sought out an ear, nose, and throat (ENT) specialist. After he examined her ears, he excused himself to consult with a neurologist by phone. When he returned, he told Michelle and Kevin that he believed the origin of her ear problem was behind the inner ear and that it involved the nerves that regulated sound. What did this mean? According to the neurologist with whom he consulted, it could be a symptom of a demyelinating disease such as multiple sclerosis (MS).

Those words fell like a guillotine. She knew what MS did to a person—she had seen it in some of her past patients. At once, her mind drifted from the conversation at hand to a memory of a patient she once knew—wheelchair bound, contracted, twisted, and unable to speak intelligible words. The patient's head had been bowed to her chest, too heavy for her neck to support. In her imagination now, Michelle was drawn to the patient's bowed head and hidden face. When at last the patient turned her head to reveal her identity, to Michelle's horror, she imagined it was her own face! The shock of imagining herself as this patient jolted her attention back to the conversation at hand. The ENT doctor was just then telling Kevin that it might not be MS, and that Michelle should be examined by a neurologist for further evaluation. Michelle agreed, and an appointment was scheduled for the following Monday.

Kevin and Michelle left the ENT physician's office with somber thoughts about what her ultimate diagnosis might involve. They decided to talk about it over lunch before returning to their apartment. Shaken by the whole experience, Michelle said, "I decided to have a lunch of vodka tonics, and only then did I feel calm." Trying to be supportive and optimistic, Kevin reminded her that she had not been diagnosed yet and that there was a chance that her symptoms were caused by a virus. He asked her not to draw any hasty conclusions until she received a firm diagnosis. Michelle saw the logic in Kevin's argument and tried not to "borrow trouble from tomorrow," as the saying goes. She accompanied Kevin home where she immediately indulged in some badly needed sleep.

Michelle went right back to work the following day. With the weekend approaching, a few more days of work would keep her busy and take her mind off her problems. However, early Saturday, Michelle suffered yet another frightening symptom—not her right ear this time, but her right eye. Her vision had become dimmed. Colors seemed to appear washed out, and pieces of written words were lost. Quite frightened, she called her ophthalmologist and met with him for an examination that afternoon.

He carefully evaluated her fully dilated eye and said that it appeared to be a case of optic neuritis. Michelle added, "He spared us the fact that this is one of the hallmark signs of multiple sclerosis." Together, Michelle and Kevin returned home after her exam and did a lot of talking and crying over the next two days. Many questions ran through her mind. "How long will I live a productive life before the ravages of the disease set in? When will my legs go?" She thought about how a disease of this kind would affect her social and recreational life with Kevin and how this would shatter their dreams of having children.

Michelle cried in disbelief. She had enjoyed such a blessed youth, then a successful professional career, and now a wonderful marriage to Kevin. She couldn't comprehend her short-lived happiness. In the legendary Camelot, the rain never fell until after sundown, but in her own Camelot, she found herself taking cover in a midday downpour of tribulation.

Corticosteroid Treatment

Finally, her Monday morning appointment with the neurologist arrived. The doctor examined her and then suggested that Michelle patiently wait to see if her symptoms resolved with time. However, Michelle and Kevin were beyond waiting any longer. They had tried that already, and her symptoms just seemed to multiply with increasing gravity. Still, the neurologist did not wish to put her through a battery of tests at this time, so he asked her to wait and watch.

Upon returning home, Michelle had a different idea. She contacted one of her physician friends who referred her to a MS specialist at Massachusetts General Hospital. The physician calmly and carefully listened to her as she related her past medical history. During this examination, he told Michelle that her condition might be a demyelinating process or, possibly, a disseminated encephalomyelitis. In either case, he had a treatment plan in mind. "None of these [diagnoses] sounded overly optimistic, but at least he had a plan. I began a treatment of eight weeks on high doses of oral [cortico]steroids," she said.

While taking the medicine, Michelle began to feel pain in her left hip. She also suffered from insomnia and experienced an increase in her appetite, both of which were common side effects of corticosteroid use. "I was a bit of a bear at home and at work, but people were accepting of me," she said. Amidst these worsening symptoms, another unexpected condition became apparent. "I was in the final stages of my prednisone taper when I found out I was pregnant...How wonderful!" she said. For Michelle, this good news was like a ray of sunlight through a cloud mass. Yet, she could not help but wonder how she would cope with the pregnancy, and at the same time, treat the symptoms of her mysterious illness. She and Kevin hoped their baby would be born healthy. Time would tell.

The following nine months seemed to pass quickly, and the only bothersome symptoms she felt during that time were a painful left hip and numbness and tingling in her hands and feet. Her vision and hearing problems seemed to improve, and the right-sided numbness she once experienced seemed to concentrate itself only around her right ribs.

In June 1992, their daughter, *Taylor*, was born. She was beautiful and appeared to be very healthy. Michelle nursed Taylor during her first few months—a difficult time for the baby because she experienced a three month period of colic. Michelle felt awful for the baby's daily episodes of acute discomfort, but eventually the colic abated, much to everyone's relief. At 13 weeks, Taylor finally established a routine pattern of sleep and wakeful periods, and so did Michelle.

Strange New Symptoms

In mid-September 1992, Michelle returned to work at Beth Israel Hospital. She felt secure in the fact that she had good childcare arranged at home for Taylor, and both she and Kevin were happily occupied with their respective jobs. A solid routine of order had been established at their home, and Michelle was optimistic about the future. Unfortunately, her illness created new challenges—most prominent at this time, severe sleep deprivation.

Her pattern of disrupted sleep first occurred in November 1992. "I'll never forget that first night I awoke at 3:30 a.m. I went to the living room couch, [and] I watched the clock all night until 7:00 a.m., time to shower for work," Michelle recalled. Much to her frustration, this aggravating condition continued for the next several months. She tried all types of over-the-counter sleep aids, but nothing worked. "I was so sleep deprived and just wanted one good night's sleep," she said.

Then in April 1993, the right-sided numbness returned, and her foot started to drag a bit as she walked. Over the next month, these symptoms worsened, and Michelle returned to her neurologist. In addition to having difficulty walking, the doctor observed that she had nystagmus and pain in the left eye, a positive Babinski reflex of the right foot, and very brisk reflexes in her right arm and leg. "To my husband and me, this was the signal of the beginning of the end," she said.

Michelle could not help but envision the progression of what she thought was the beginning of MS—first a cane, then a wheelchair, and ultimately confinement to a death bed. The neurologist offered to treat her with another course of oral prednisone, but she refused because she thought that the steroids might contribute to further sleep deprivation. She went home without any prescription drugs, and she waited. After about one month, her condition of chronic insomnia mysteriously ceased without any medical intervention. Michelle wondered what kind of illness would produce such intermittent and transient neurologic symptoms. From a nurse's perspective, her symptoms were unlike any she had ever encountered in her career. Yet, she knew she wasn't imagining these things, so what was happening?

All in my Head

The summer of 1993 passed without major incidence, but also without notable improvement. Then around September, Michelle noticed a troublesome pattern of forgetfulness. For someone who was once a fluent educator, she now struggled to think of the words she wanted to speak. What was going on? Not only did she have word retrieval difficulties, but she felt exhausted and depleted of all energy. She prayed that these symptoms would be self-resolving as some of the others had been.

Anxiety was also becoming a problem. She had noticed it starting to build over the past few months. Then one Saturday morning in November, Michelle was awakened at 4:00 a.m. by an overwhelming feeling of dread—a panic attack. Taylor was crying in her crib, but Michelle just lay in bed unresponsive to her cries. Michelle pulled the covers tightly over her head, unable to deal emotionally with duties she once found pleasurable. Kevin wasn't sure exactly what was happening to his wife, but he got up and took care of Taylor. He was very concerned about Michelle—he had never seen her immobilized by anxiety like this before.

Both Kevin and Michelle knew she needed to consult with a psychiatrist soon—the sooner the better. Michelle said, "I knew that I had to see someone professional that day to reassure myself that I wasn't crazy." Fortunately, the psychiatrist she contacted had an opening that afternoon, and he agreed to meet with her to discuss her worsening state of anxiety. Kevin accompanied her to the appointment. The soft-spoken physician invited the couple to take a seat and tell him about themselves and the history of Michelle's anxieties. He eventually asked her if she felt depressed.

Through a stream of tears, Michelle answered, "No, I'm not depressed. I have a wonderful husband, a beautiful daughter, the best job anyone could want, and a full life ahead of me." He gently suggested to her that, perhaps, she was suffering from depression without knowing it. This suggestion seemed plausible to Michelle, and she eventually agreed to try an antidepressant medication that he recommended. It worked for her depression but not for her anxiety, so he later prescribed an anxiolytic (anti-anxiety drug). With the addition of this medicine, her state of mind improved, and she was able to function much better at home and at work.

The Stork Revisits

From November 1993 until May 1994, Michelle noticed improvements both emotionally and physically. She was so relieved and wondered if her three year struggle with this strange illness was finally abating. That optimism turned out to be premature because May brought a resurgence of painful symptoms. She recalled, "The buzzing band around my right thorax came back with a vengeance. The burning pain was terrible. I also found out around this time that I was pregnant. My due date was November 20, 1994."

Michelle tolerated her symptoms during her pregnancy, but in August 1994, just as she entered her third trimester, she experienced a second episode of meningitis. "I had all the same symptoms as I had had in New Mexico [in 1991], except my fever spiked to 104 degrees, and I didn't always know where I was." Another spinal tap revealed an elevated white blood cell count of 121, a low-normal level of spinal fluid glucose, and normal levels of protein.

She remained in the hospital for a short time while the doctors monitored the baby's health and her own. Happily, the baby had gained two pounds by the time Michelle was discharged. On the other hand, Michelle had lost 11 pounds because she was unable to eat anything except an occasional vanilla shake. Still, she was happy to be going home and hoped the meningitis would resolve quickly.

Two weeks after returning home, that hope was dashed when she was readmitted to the hospital. A new spinal tap showed that her white blood count had risen to 158. Since viral meningitis is treated primarily with rest and usually resolves with time, and this is what the doctors suspected, Michelle chose to return home and treat her fever with Motrin and eat home cooked meals. "I stayed at home for a couple of weeks until the symptoms got worse again," she said. Once again, she returned to the hospital where a fourth spinal tap was performed. It showed that her white blood count had risen to 326, and that she also had an elevated spinal fluid protein.

Blood was drawn, and tests confirmed that her serum had elevations in white blood cells, platelets, and sed rate. "I clearly had some infection going on, but they were unable to find it," Michelle noted. Interestingly, at this point in time, samples of her blood and spinal fluid were tested for Lyme disease using the enzyme linked immunosorbent assay (ELISA). It was the first time that Lyme disease had been suspected as a possible cause of her apparent infection. However, that possibility was ruled out when the ELISA results came back negative.

This second bout of meningitis resolved completely within the next month. Still, Michelle and Kevin knew the battle with her mysterious illness was likely to wage on, so they decided to hire a nanny to help Michelle with Taylor and their second baby. The nanny they hired was *Karen* from Scotland, a kind and sensible 20 year old, who became a real asset to the family. With Karen's help and the availability of two sets of grandparents, Michelle and Kevin had adequate help for the children. Exactly one week after Karen's arrival, Michelle gave birth to their second baby, *John*.

After three months at home with baby John and Taylor, Michelle returned to work. She noticed that she didn't have the get-up-and-go she once had, but she was excited to return to work nonetheless. "I did very well over the next five months, with the only exception being lack of sleep. This never [reverted] back to anything you could call normal," she said.

Meningitis—A Third Bout

In April 1995, Michelle was admitted to the hospital again—this time with a third case of meningitis. Tests were performed with the following results: enterovirus polymerase chain reaction (PCR) was negative, and herpes simplex virus (HSV) titers were also negative. Both the treating doctor and Michelle's neurologist were perplexed over the cause of her repeated cases of meningitis. Referring back to earlier MRIs, the doctors concurred that no lesions were present to indicate MS, and no oligoclonal banding (marker that suggests inflammation of the central nervous system) was found in Michelle's spinal fluid. Since evidence was lacking for a firm MS diagnosis, the doctors agreed to give her symptoms a temporary explanation, atypical MS and Mollaret's meningitis. Michelle was puzzled over the latter diagnosis because her spinal fluid did not show any evidence of Mollaret's cells. Now, she thought, her illness was just about as mysterious as the diagnoses she had been given.

Throughout the following year of 1996, Michelle experienced an ongoing series of ailments, including frequent sore throats, eye pain, ear pain, light sensitivity, severe headaches, jaw pain, and muscle pains. None of her physicians understood why she was suffering with these strange and seemingly unrelated symptoms. Needless to say, Michelle felt very helpless despite having access to what she thought was the best medical care a patient could possibly want.

In September 1996, amidst all of these painful

symptoms, Michelle learned that she was expecting their third child, due the following June. This was welcome news but spawned obvious concerns. Would this baby be healthy if she continued to experience these painful symptoms? Could she endure this pregnancy without getting adequate sleep? Lack of sleep was still an ongoing and aggravating problem for Michelle, and it had been so for the past three years. At long last, she decided to see a sleep specialist at Massachusetts General Hospital.

At the doctor's suggestion, Michelle underwent an overnight sleep study which revealed that she had moderately disruptive limb movements that prevented her from reaching deeper stages of sleep. A variety of sleep medications were prescribed, but none of them proved helpful. Finally, a Duragesic patch was prescribed, but after the third day, her speech slurred so badly that she immediately removed the patch. Frustrated, Michelle said, "I had no problems falling asleep. I just could not stay asleep past 3 or 4 a.m." Understandably, she became increasingly irritable from lack of sleep, so she decided to try a short-acting, antianxiety medication when she woke in the early morning hours. This seemed to remedy the problem for a while.

Corticosteroids Again

In June of 1997, Michelle gave birth to her third baby, *Phil*. "I did fine postpartum until December 1997. At this time, I was admitted to the hospital after six weeks of left eye pain, light sensitivity, right leg numbness, and a crawling sensation in my skin," she said. When she spoke to the doctor, she explained that three days prior to this, she had experienced an onslaught of other very odd symptoms, including urinary urgency, incontinence, sore throat, neck soreness and pain, chills, night sweats, feeling feverish despite no measurable fever, and slowness of speech. A lumbar puncture was done, but it showed nothing abnormal, so the neurologist thought perhaps she was experiencing a flare up of MS symptoms. The doctor ordered intravenous (IV) therapy of methylprednisolone on a tapering dose over the next nine days. Three of those days were supervised by the doctor while Michelle remained in the hospital, and after her discharge home, Michelle finished the IV therapy there.

Corticosteroids, such as methylprednisolone and prednisone, are powerful drugs that have a suppressive effect on immune function. The use of these drugs can result in an increased susceptibility to infections or can make an existing infection spread and become more fully entrenched and more difficult to deal with and treat.

One day after finishing the IV therapy, Michelle was back in the hospital with severely aggravated symptoms. She presented with severe muscle pain, nausea, lower abdominal pain, migrating joint pains, a burning sensation of her tongue, hair loss, burning and painful bumps on her scalp, urinary and fecal incontinence, light sensitivity, neck stiffness, and an overall feeling of burning skin.

Tests were performed immediately. An abdominal scan was negative. Blood tests showed an elevation in white blood cells, neutrophils, and absolute neutrophils. Her lymphocytes were low as well as one of her liver functions. The doctor gave her a diagnosis of "post viral syndrome." She was discharged home without treatment and advised to follow up with her neurologist as soon as possible. Michelle wondered what kind of virus would cause these awful symptoms. "I was scared to death not knowing what was wrong with me," she said.

Process of Elimination

In January 1998, Kevin accompanied Michelle to her follow-up visit with the neurologist. This time they wanted some answers that made sense. Frustrated, Michelle said, "I really had not felt well in over six months, and it wasn't just MS symptoms or meningitis. I felt as though my body was toxic and something was making me incredibly sick." The doctor considered other causes for her condition and suggested that perhaps she had a connective tissue disease. Blood was drawn to test for lupus, rheumatoid factor, the sed rate (to evaluate inflammation), and a complete blood count. Everything was normal except for low counts on both hemoglobin and hematocrit.

Michelle's primary doctor and her neurologist cooperated in an effort to begin ruling out possible causes for her many and varied symptoms. The brain MRI that was performed revealed no lesions. An electromyelogram was conducted for vasculitis and peripheral neuropathy, and those results were also negative. Michelle pressed her physicians to determine a single diagnosis that might be the cause of all these symptoms, but they felt one explanation was highly unlikely. In fact, after all these tests were performed, any firm diagnosis still eluded them, and Michelle was still suffering.

Then in April 1998, Michelle woke in the middle of the night with excruciating pain in her right knee. It persisted through the following day. "I was taking Motrin as though it was candy," she recalled. Her knee became noticeably swollen in front and behind the knee, and when she walked on it, it sounded "crunchy." She immediately arranged an appointment with a rheumatologist, and he examined her knee.

He confirmed what she already knew—the knee was swollen and exhibited crepitus (crunchy sound when moved)—and considered performing a tap of the fluid surrounding the knee. The procedure was not carried out because of insufficient fluid, and so he advised her to go home and watch the knee. If the knee became more swollen, then he would perform a tap and analyze the fluid at that time. As it turned out, this symptom was just as transient as many of the previous ones, and she never needed to return to this rheumatologist.

A Colleague's Nephew

During the spring of 1998, a hospital colleague with whom Michelle shared an office, mentioned that her nephew had symptoms like Michelle's, and he had been diagnosed with Lyme disease. Michelle explained that she had been tested for the disease before, but the ELISA results were negative. Her colleague mentioned that her nephew also tested negative for Lyme, yet he still had the disease. This piqued Michelle's curiosity. She wondered if she had Lyme disease all this time, too, despite negative test results. At Michelle's request, her friend provided the name of a Lyme disease specialist with whom she socialized, and Michelle made an appointment for the following week.

Hopeful that she might be on the right track at last, Michelle went home to do some research on the disease over the Internet. She found a website that listed possible symptoms commonly associated with Lyme disease, and she was shocked. "I had close to every symptom listed on this one particular website. I also found information that stated you needn't test positive for Lyme to have the disease. Maybe this is what I had," she said.

In preparation for her consultation with the Lyme disease doctor in Boston, she prepared a package to send to him in advance of her appointment. In it she put all her past medical records and a 12 page write-up of the last eight years of symptoms, ruled-out diagnoses, and hospitalizations. She also included a classic article from a respected scientific journal that discussed case histories where Lyme disease patients had experienced the associated triad of meningitis, cranial neuritis (inflammation of one or more cranial nerves), and radiculoneuritis (peripheral neuropathy and spinal nerve pain)—just like she had experienced.

Saying Goodbye

In April, Michelle experienced another bout of debilitating symptoms, including memory loss and mental "fog," and was barely able to perform her duties at work without resting. "The physician that I worked with knew that I was having a very hard time. He insisted that I take at least a one hour nap after lunch so I could regain my strength and make it through the rest of the day," she explained. The doctor volunteered to see Michelle's patients during the afternoon while she rested. "We were a true team. God, how I miss that!" Michelle said sadly.

Facing the reality of her illness, she decided she had no choice but to resign from the profession she loved so dearly. She had worked as long as she possibly could without feeling that she might be putting a patient at risk by making some medication error. The disease had begun to affect her brain, and at this point, she did what any responsible nurse would do—resign.

On her last day at work, her colleagues presented her with a very special kind of gift that is given only to those resigning from high posts at the hospital—a beautiful rocking chair. Michelle was deeply touched by this gesture of sincere appreciation. "I was so honored and so touched. No one can imagine how much," she said.

Leaving a profession she loved so much was emotionally shattering. "I could not have been more devastated. I had wanted to be a nurse my whole life and could not have been happier in my present position. I was so honored to receive my Harvard/Beth Israel Hospital chair," she said as tears welled up in her eyes.

Her early retirement was one of the most costly

sacrifices she could have made. Her work was part of her personal identity. What would she do without this occupation to bring her personal satisfaction and intellectual challenge? Kevin tried to reassure her, "Now you can be a full-time mother and stay at home." She didn't think he understood the devastation she felt. "No one will ever understand how hard that was for me," she said. Now without work obligations, Michelle concentrated even harder on regaining good health. She hoped that perhaps one day, she could return to her nursing profession.

Lyme Specialist

Michelle was looking forward to her appointment with the Lyme disease doctor, and Kevin agreed to accompany her. When they met with the physician, they spoke for two hours about her medical history. He read over the papers she had sent to him and asked her some questions. At the conclusion of the interview, Michelle waited quietly for his professional opinion. Then he said, "I seriously doubt it is Lyme disease because (1) you never tested positive for Lyme; (2) you didn't have a Lyme rash confirmed by a doctor, so we don't know what kind of rash you had; and (3) you had this rash in January [which is] not a time we [typically] see Lyme disease rashes."

In utter shock, Michelle said, "But what about all the symptoms I have: joint pain, swelling, cranial nerve damage, spinal cord damage, and all the bouts of meningitis? Here is the paper written about this triad of symptoms." The doctor repeated, "You have never tested positive for Lyme, so I don't think that is what you have."

Michelle left the office in deep despair. She knew that this doctor was simply wrong. Kevin's opinion was that the doctor was the specialist, and he ought to know whether or not this case sounded like Lyme disease. He placed his faith in this authority's opinion, and so he accepted it without question. Conversely, Michelle was very disturbed by his conclusions, and she was going to go back to her neurologist to get another referral to a different Lyme disease doctor.

When she met with the neurologist, he tried to discourage her from pursuing her seemingly unfounded medical theory. He thought she was wasting time inquiring about a disease that he felt had nothing to do with her ailments. Although he admitted that MS alone would not account for all of her bizarre symptoms, he speculated that she actually suffered from two disorders concurrently, MS and fibromyalgia. Michelle did not buy into this explanation and begged him to refer her to another Lyme disease doctor. He finally decided to refer her to a neurologic Lyme specialist located on the western part of Long Island, New York.

Strike Two

Together, Kevin and Michelle drove for four hours to her appointment on Long Island. After the physician examined her and discussed her history, he also concluded that she did not have Lyme disease for the same reasons cited by the first Lyme specialist she consulted. Instead, he did say that she might have neuro-Behcet's syndrome. The doctor explained, "It's a disease most often found in Iranian men, but it can occur in other people. Your neurologic symptoms, plus the eye pain, makes me want to rule this out. I will speak to your neurologist about this."

Michelle could not believe what she had just heard—a disease most often found in Iranian men! She could not understand why these experts would so easily rule out the much more likely Lyme disease in favor of a very rare disorder. She explained, "When you read the CDC guidelines for diagnosing Lyme disease, they specifically state that it is a clinical diagnosis with support from the blood work." She felt frustrated because she thought that her current condition and her medical history showed overwhelming clinical evidence of Lyme disease.

When she left the doctor's office, she sat on one of the benches outside the clinic and waited for Kevin to get the car and pick her up. As she contemplated what had just transpired inside, she began to cry hysterically. Twice she had consulted with Lyme disease specialists who ruled out Lyme based on one test result only. Where could she find knowledgeable help? How long would that take and at what cost to Michelle's body and mind?

Kevin approached Michelle and helped her into the car. He tried to reason with her, "How many Lyme experts can be wrong? Haven't we seen enough?" He could not understand why Michelle held so strongly to the opinion that she had Lyme disease when two specialists had ruled it out.

When they returned home, Michelle immediately made a call to her neurologist to tell him what the Lyme doctor had concluded. He said to her, "Well, Michelle, will you agree with me to finally put this Lyme disease thing to rest?" She did not answer that question because she believed the infection was being dismissed without a rational justification and that these two doctors, along with her neurologist, refused to think beyond one test result. She reasoned to herself, "I did not believe I had an absolutely obscure disease of Iranian men! My symptoms didn't fit that diagnosis, but they sure fit Lyme disease."

Local Support Group

After returning home, Michelle found a listing in the local paper for a Lyme disease support group, and she decided to attend the next meeting. "I learned more about the trouble with diagnosing Lyme disease in that one hour than I had ever heard from any doctor," said Michelle. She also learned about how divided the medical community was over how to diagnose and treat the illness.

Lyme disease can be misdiagnosed as other diseases. Three of the ten people Michelle met at the support group meeting had been previously diagnosed with MS before they learned they had Lyme disease. She thought about how many years she might have had this disease and hoped it wasn't too late to gain back a measure of good health. After attending this meeting, she was even more convinced that she had been misdiagnosed with MS and fibromyalgia. Her search for a knowledgeable doctor continued as she faced autumn, the most difficult time of the year in terms of her health.

The approaching fall of 1998 was a predictably hard one. "For some reason, this particular time of year has always been the worst as far as how I feel," she related. This year was no different. During the months of September through December, she saw three doctors for more painful symptoms, and she was hospitalized one day before Thanksgiving.

At the hospital, she presented with the same combination of weird symptoms, including horrible headaches, left eye pain, ear infections, sore throat, hair loss, weight gain, scalp pain, extreme fatigue, muscle pain, joint aches, strange rashes, right foot drop, and right leg weakness. In addition to these symptoms, she also had blood in her urine. The hospital tested her urine for bacteria, but the results were negative.

Testing Endurance

Michelle and Kevin were becoming emotionally overwhelmed. They had been subjected to such a medical runaround that it was exasperating, to say the least. Recalling how her illness and the frustration with numerous doctors affected their marriage and family, Michelle said, "Kevin, who had been such a strong support for me in the beginning, was now getting apathetic. My parents were up in Vermont sending me Mass cards from their church, but my youngest brother was still there for me when I needed to talk with someone."

Clearly, Michelle's ongoing medical dilemma over the past eight years had made some in her family feel helpless, and they were showing the effects. Kevin's endurance as her advocate and caregiver was waning. It seemed as though nothing he did helped his wife get well. He always had faith in the medical system of which his wife was once a member. Now that she was a patient, that system seemed a frustrating maze of specialists with no real answers. In his profession, Kevin was accustomed to relying on the expertise and educated opinions of authorities such as physicians. As a patient advocate, he now began to realize that medical professionals are not necessarily as knowledgeable as commonly believed.

The doctors simply did not know what was wrong with Michelle, and they put her through many questionable tests and exhibited little empathy. When it appeared as though a doctor knew what was wrong, Michelle disagreed. Kevin was tired. He tried to find help for Michelle, to be her protector and advocate, but he was not prepared for this long and frustrating battle. He felt he was no longer helpful to her personally, so he resorted to helping in the only way he could see direct benefit—caring for the children and being a reliable provider.

Obviously, emotional and psychological assets were stretched to their limits. That's just the point—all advocates, caregivers, and support networks have their limits. That is why so many patients with chronic illnesses feel they are fighting the battle all alone. For Michelle, her family support was eroding with the passage of time, but it was never gone completely. She was never left without at least one person she could lean on during those challenging times—she just wanted that person to always be Kevin. In the final analysis, she realized that if she was going to get better, she had to rely upon her own assets, her nursing education, and common sense. She listened to her own body and did not allow anyone to dissuade her from what she knew and felt was happening to that body. She was solely in charge of her healthcare.

It was difficult for her, and she felt very depressed at times. "I felt like a constant complainer, and the people around me were growing weary of hearing it," she said. After going on so many unproductive doctor appointments, listening to so many opinions—some of which sounded logical to Kevin, but not to Michelle—Kevin was just burned out. He decided that after this, he would only accompany her on visits he thought were important. He could not be absent from his job for every consultation. How long would his employer accept absences that did not result in some headway anyway? Kevin had responsibilities to his law firm and to his family as their main bread winner, so he made some difficult choices.

As for Michelle, she felt resentment at what she perceived as his emotional abandonment of her. However, as the patient, she had to work at getting better—that was truly *her* job. Her husband would be sitting on the sidelines, but she had to stay in the game. She had no choice. Logically, she knew they were both reacting to extraordinary stress. As a nurse, though, she also knew that when hardships are faced head on as a family unit, the family benefits and so does the patient. *That wasn't happening here*, she thought. Kevin wasn't going to be there for her in the way that she thought he would be. She missed his support and comfort, but she understood that he was doing all that he could. It was a truth that was hard to accept.

Infectious Disease Doctor

During the winter of 1998-1999, Michelle saw an infectious disease doctor who thought that her symptoms might be a disorder called Whipple's disease. Michelle endured a complete gastrointestinal work-up, but the results proved negative. The doctor then ordered a repeat of a cervical MRI, and her report noted, "a small area of hyperintensity on long TR images at the level of C2 (second cervical vertebra). Its appearance is totally nonspecific. It certainly could represent an MS plaque, though I do not see any abnormalities in the cervical cord."

Michelle's neurologist scheduled another brain MRI for Michelle, and, once again, it showed no abnormalities. After all the tests were performed, the neurologist held to the opinion that Michelle had multiple sclerosis with some other (undiagnosed) process going on. Michelle, however, would not accept that explanation.

Then in March, a very troubling symptom appeared—one that frightened Michelle more than any of the others she had previously experienced. "[I was having] problems concentrating, finding the right names for objects, and forgetting what I did two minutes earlier. The physical problems were one issue, but please, don't take away my ability to communicate with the world," she said.

Once, as an example, she was trying to describe a kite to her two-year-old son, but the right word would not come to mind. Instead she stuttered, "Look at the diamond, tail thing with the thread." Incredibly frustrated over her lack of mental clarity and language command, she remained isolated at home so that others would not notice her newest handicap.

This self-imposed isolation was disturbing, but as the year 1999 passed, more and more of her friends distanced themselves from her. "Friends began to stop asking how I was because there was never any good news, and I didn't blame them one bit. But my family stopped asking, too, and this really hurt." Kevin was likewise discouraged over her chronic poor health. If the doctors weren't sure what was wrong with her, how could he understand it? How could he give a satisfying reply to those who asked about Michelle?

As time passed, he began to withdraw from Michelle and communicated only sparingly. "I no longer got words of encouragement from him. I would beg for a hug! After two years of marriage counseling, we have both come to realize [that] we are doing what we were each capable of [doing]. I felt quite abandoned," she said.

Angry at the medical community for her present state of health, Michelle said, "What had happened to me was not my fault!" With legitimate reason for complaint, she adamantly blamed the doctors she consulted for not finding the correct diagnosis earlier. Now she feared there was little hope that she would ever be cured.

The children began to wonder the same. They often asked their mother, "What were you like before you got sick, Mom?" She explained that she did a lot of skiing, enjoyed playing basketball, and often beat their dad at tennis. They marveled as they envisioned her doing those things, and they laughed when she related how much she loved to plan elaborate parties and be the last person to leave a gathering. As their laughter waned, their thoughts were directed back to the real question, "What is wrong with you, Mom?" Michelle had to hide her emotions to answer that question. She knew that the children needed to hear something encouraging. "We haven't figured it out yet, but we will soon, and then I'll be okay," she reassured them.

A Florida Clinic

Michelle wanted nothing more than to have some doctor "figure this out," and soon, because her children had never known a healthy mother. More than anything else, she wanted to be the active mother and wife she was supposed to be, that she knew she could be. Nine years had passed since she experienced her first symptoms of this illness—when were things going to get better?

In January 2000, her neurologist contacted a neuro-Behcet's specialist who practiced at a well-known clinic in Jacksonville, Florida. An appointment was scheduled for Michelle, and Kevin took a week off from work to accompany her there. During the meeting, the doctor looked over the notes from Michelle's neurologist and said, "I seriously doubt you have neuro-Behcet's." Kevin and Michelle looked at each other in amazement and wanted to know why they were told to travel this distance to meet with him if neuro-Behcet's could be ruled out simply by reviewing medical records.

Observing their irritation over the time, effort, and money spent to be present at this appointment, the doctor said, "Well, since you are here, we may as well do a work-up of your symptoms and see what we come up with." The specialist estimated that Michelle's tests would extend into the following week. Kevin had to return to his job in Boston and couldn't stay the entire time, so Michelle kept a room at a nearby hotel and planned to return home by herself.

During the first week while Kevin was still there, Michelle was examined by three different specialists, a neurologist who specialized in migraines, a rheumatologist, and an infectious disease physician. Many tests were performed, including blood work and an MRI of the brain and spine. The tests revealed "significant anemia, increased anticardiolipin antibodies, an increase in A1 globulin, and a decrease in C3 and C4 complement levels."

The final test was performed while Kevin was gone and one day prior to Michelle's departure for home. It was performed by a urologist, the fourth doctor on Michelle's list of physicians from this clinic. This test was called the bladder distention test, and general anesthesia was necessary, something previous tests did not employ. The object of this test was to evaluate whether or not she had interstitial cystitis (inflammation of the bladder wall). The procedure went smoothly, but the next morning when she awoke in her hotel room, something was terribly wrong.

"As I was getting out of bed, I noticed that it was next to impossible to bend my legs in any fashion. It felt as though they were locked at the knee," Michelle explained. She called the urologist, and he urged her to go to the emergency room (ER) without delay. Michelle could barely walk, let alone drive herself to an ER. Finally, with the help of hotel staff, she was pushed in a hotel wheelchair, ushered into a cab, and was delivered to the emergency room for examination.

The ER doctors said that her locked legs were probably the result of a reaction to the general anesthesia from the day before. To counteract this adverse reaction, she was given IV Valium which ultimately worked. Five hours later, she left the emergency room in a wheelchair for her discharge evaluation with the neuro-Behcet's specialist at the clinic.

Discharge Diagnosis

In the final analysis, Lyme disease, rheumatoid arthritis, and multiple sclerosis were simply ruled out. The specialist could not offer any explanation for the type of disease that would cause all of Michelle's symptoms. However, he did give her some personal advice before her discharge. He said, "Mrs. O'Leary, while it is true that we have not been able to find out specifically what it is you have, I suggest that you try to stop being a wimp and tough things out for the sake of your family."

Amazed at his derisive attitude and disgusted over his grossly inaccurate assessment of her medical circumstances, she said to him, "If I were your wife or sister and came to you for help in figuring out what I had, would you still call me a wimp? You are the most unprofessional doctor I have ever met, and this is not the last you will hear from me. Because you can't figure out what I have does not make me a wimp, but perhaps it makes you incompetent." That said, she abruptly turned her wheelchair and rolled out of his office.

Michelle made her way to the airport to catch a flight back to Boston. By then, her leg spasms had finally relaxed, and she could navigate without a wheelchair. On the plane, she quietly cried. She didn't know what she was going to do now. She had been hospitalized, evaluated, and tested by many different specialists, and still no one knew what was wrong with her. The doctors either washed their hands of her or resorted to blaming her for overreacting to her aches and pains. They weren't the only ones who were frustrated over the years she had spent searching in vain for a diagnosis and treatment. "So many people were giving up. My husband came to [fewer and fewer] appointments, [and] it was getting harder to [deal] with the fatigue and the confusion. My parents continued to pray, but what I really needed was help and a hug!" she confessed.

When she returned home, she met with her neurologist, and together they reviewed the test results from the Florida trip. He was also desperately seeking an explanation for her degenerative condition and had come up with one more idea. He wanted to test her for something called Mediterranean fever. Michelle thought to herself, "Now we were going from the ridiculous to the sublime! I had had enough." She realized then that it was up to her to decipher where in this process the specialists had gone wrong. They missed something, and she had to backtrack and find it.

Lyme Specialist #3

Thinking back on the various doctors she had consulted and what had been ruled out so far, Michelle decided to return to the local Lyme disease support group and talk to the support group leader. To Michelle, this seemed the most logical place to start over again on her own investigation.

As she began to relate her circumstances to the group's president, Michelle explained how her doctors thought she had atypical MS with another ongoing process, perhaps fibromyalgia. When the leader shared the name of her own Lyme doctor, she explained that many people who used antibiotics or immune suppressive corticosteroids prior to, or at the time of testing, could test negative for Lyme. This information grabbed Michelle's attention because she had initially been treated with corticosteroids.

She returned home and told Kevin what she learned and that she wanted to consult with a new Lyme specialist—a third one. He accompanied her to the appointment, and they took with them a growing file of medical records. The doctor spent two hours interviewing Michelle and examining her. He explained that before he would give his opinion, he wanted to run a few tests, and he would call her within two weeks. She agreed to this plan, and blood was drawn for testing.

Two weeks passed, four weeks passed, and then two and a half months passed, and still nothing came from the doctor's office except bills. Finally, Michelle sent a letter to the doctor's office inquiring about her test results. Two days later, when Michelle was sitting outside on her back porch, the phone rang. It was the Lyme disease doctor calling to apologize for the delay in getting back to her with the test results. He had them in hand now, and after a short pause, he interpreted the report. He said, "Yes, indeed, you have Lyme disease. The test results came back strongly positive." A long, overdue calmness overshadowed her. It was relief along with vindication at last! Now she had one more obvious question to ask the doctor—why did her past test results come back negative if she had Lyme disease all along?

He explained that the two-tiered testing procedure that is commonly employed by doctors for Lyme disease is flawed. When a patient presents with clinical evidence of Lyme disease, or if Lyme disease is suspected, the doctor will have blood drawn for an ELISA (antibody test). If this test comes back positive, then the more comprehensive Western blot tests are performed. Conversely, if the ELISA comes back negative—which it frequently does—then the doctor will not feel justified in writing an order for a Western blot. Many doctors rely too heavily upon the results of the less accurate ELISA and prematurely rule out a Lyme diagnosis. This restrictive approach, accepted by the majority of physicians, often results in missed Lyme disease diagnoses, allowing patients to unwittingly become chronic sufferers— perhaps for years, like Michelle.

The physician then outlined an antibiotic therapy protocol for Michelle and asked for her pharmacy information. He added that no follow-up appointment was necessary since he communicated with his patients over the Internet and by phone. Any adjustment to the treatment regimen was made in this manner. Michelle was very hesitant about committing herself to his care after he revealed this information. She said, "I was not at all sure that this was the type of physician I wanted to treat me for my Lyme disease." She told the doctor she would have to think about it and get back to him later.

After she hung up the phone, she put her head in her hands and began to cry. Following nearly 10 years of fighting an elusive disease, she had every right to release her emotions. A firm diagnosis had been established, yet she still could not begin treatment. She wondered why every effort she made was met with some new roadblock. Enough of that now! She wiped her eyes and immediately called one of her dear friends to invite her over to the house to celebrate the diagnostic news.

Her friend came by with a bottle of wine, and they drank and talked about Michelle's future after her recovery. It was great to imagine herself cured and enjoying life again after losing a decade of her life to this illness. She had a lot to catch up on with Kevin—how she missed the happiness they shared, once upon a time, long ago and far away in their own private Camelot.

When Michelle called Kevin at the office to tell him the doctor's news, the secretary told her that he was in a conference and would have to return her call. When he finally did, Michelle excitedly told him that her test results were positive. Naturally, Kevin was skeptical and had many of the same questions Michelle had initially. She reminded him that for the past two years, she suspected Lyme but had failed to find someone who could support it with blood tests. Now she also knew why.

Despite this, Kevin remained reservedly cautious about accepting this doctor's Lyme disease diagnosis—one he knew Michelle was hoping to get one day. Michelle explained to Kevin that this Lyme doctor was also treating another person, who like herself, had been previously misdiagnosed with fibromyalgia for three years. Michelle was disappointed over Kevin's initial reservations, but she realized that he needed time to digest this new information before they discussed it again.

Meanwhile, Michelle had to continue her pursuit of a knowledgeable doctor to properly treat her now that she was on the right track. She had no idea, then, that this was not going to be an easy task. The reason why would ultimately alarm and enrage her as a healthcare consumer.

The Monkey in the Middle

Michelle again contacted the head of the local Lyme support group and related her recent experience with the latest Lyme disease doctor. She also explained her hesitation over being treated by a doctor without the advantages associated with personal follow-up consultations. Michelle asked the woman if she could recommend any other practitioners. She gave Michelle two other names—one was a nurse practitioner and the other a physician—but neither practiced in Massachusetts.

"I soon found out why no one went to see the Lyme specialists in Massachusetts. It appeared as though the specialists in Massachusetts only treated Lyme disease for two to four weeks, even though the patient may have had the disease for years," Michelle explained. Learning about the medical community's division over treatment protocols came as an eye opener to Michelle, who had once been a faithful member of the healthcare system. "One camp believes that all cases of Lyme disease can be cured by two to four weeks of antibiotics, while the opposite camp believes that Lyme disease should be treated until symptoms are gone," she explained.

She also learned that some Lyme disease doctors, who have treated patients with long-term antibiotics, have had their medical practices threatened; others have backed away from open-ended treatment because of that knowledge. Michelle commented, "Never has medicine seen such a divide nor such drastic steps been taken to fight a philosophical difference as to how to treat Lyme disease. This divide should be fought in clinical trials to determine if long-term treatment is beneficial or not, not in the court of law. The patient is the monkey in the middle having to decide which camp [he] thinks is right."

The first hurdle—getting a competent Lyme disease diagnosis—is difficult enough. Attempting to find open-ended treatment—treatment until symptoms are gone—is the next significant challenge. The patient must navigate a system that is dominated by restrictive guidelines that encourage dropping legitimate cases prematurely, both in diagnosis and during treatment. Michelle wondered if she would be able to find effective treatment amidst all this political hullabaloo.

Competent Diagnosis and Treatment

The first thing she had to do was make a personal choice in this issue, and she decided that she wanted to be treated until her symptoms were gone. After making that decision, she then made an appointment with the nurse practitioner (NP) recommended by the Lyme support group president. Incidentally, the NP was in practice with a pediatric Lyme disease specialist at the time.

After Michelle's examination and interview, the clinician ordered a series of diagnostic tests including cervical and thoracic MRIs, a brain SPECT scan, a spinal tap, and additional blood tests. The MRIs revealed damage to the spinal cord. "This accounted for the numbness, tingling, foot drop, bowel and bladder incontinence, eye pain, and rib soreness," Michelle said.

The brain SPECT scan also revealed abnormalities— "a heterogeneous decrease in blood flow throughout the cerebral cortex." This condition could explain her episodes of mental fog and poor memory recall. Michelle's blood was also tested for other infections, and the results showed that she had three: ehrlichiosis, babesiosis, and bartonella (cat scratch disease). All three would need to be treated as well as Borrelia burgdorferi (Bb), the causative agent of Lyme disease.

Due to the severity of the damage to Michelle's spinal cord, the NP decided to start her on IV therapy. A PICC line was threaded up her arm toward her chest, and it was something that felt very cumbersome at first. "But I soon got the hang of wearing the proper clothes to cover the intravenous catheter. I was taught how to maintain the line and how to change the bag of antibiotics daily. It soon became very routine," Michelle said.

Time to Reflect

Michelle had a lot of time now to think about the past ten years—and where she might have contracted Lyme disease. Admittedly, she had been to every endemic region in the Northeast, so she could have been exposed at any of these locations. However, considering the timeline of her medical history, one place stood out as the most likely. She explained, "The fall before my symptoms started, we had spent a long weekend in Fairfield, Connecticut, visiting friends. It was about 1½ months after that, that I had these ringworm-like rashes on the back of my neck."

One might think that Michelle's nursing background would have expedited a proper diagnosis. However, she admitted that Lyme disease never came to mind. After all, she was a diabetes nurse specialist dedicated solely to that field. She hadn't even considered Lyme disease as a cause for her illness until two years before the diagnosis. Like other members of the medical community, she trusted in the expertise of other specialists to discover the cause of her illness.

She had no idea then about the arguable two-tiered testing protocol that is relied upon to screen Lyme disease. Consequently, she had no reason to question whenever a specialist reported negative test results for Lyme. She didn't realize that being tested after taking corticosteroids or antibiotics might produce a false negative test result. She simply did not know these things.

Her acquaintance with the local Lyme disease group in 1998 was her educational introduction to Lyme disease. Ever since then, she held to the underlying belief that Lyme disease was the most probable cause of her illness. She wasted no time and consulted not one, but three physicians who called themselves Lyme disease specialists. She learned the hard way that most physicians operate according to very rigid guidelines for diagnosis and treatment of the illness. Despite this, she did not give up. She continued her search for a clinician whose knowledge extended beyond the guidelines that are popularly held.

Three months after receiving her Lyme disease and co-infection diagnosis, she began IV therapy. It was a long struggle, but she was finally where she needed to be. She was relieved that now she could concentrate on her recovery. She was excited about what that would ultimately mean for her relationship with Kevin and the children.

Pediatric Help

At Michelle's two month follow-up appointment, she had an opportunity to speak with the pediatric Lyme disease specialist about some odd symptoms that her children exhibited. She explained that she had undiagnosed Lyme disease during each of her three pregnancies and wondered if her children might also have this illness.

She explained that when she was carrying Taylor, she was on a 20 mg taper of prednisone, prescribed as treatment for symptoms of multiple sclerosis. At the age of three, Taylor started showing significant aggression toward other children. At age seven, she had been diagnosed with ADHD along with a nonverbal learning disorder. Even though she was now eight years old, Taylor's social and emotional problems persisted.

During Michelle's third trimester of her pregnancy with their son, John, she experienced a serious bout of meningitis accompanied by high fevers. Early on, John had swollen kidneys, but that resolved, and he never had problems with this condition again. At the age of two, however, Michelle and Kevin noticed that John was unusually clumsy—even falling down on level surfaces without apparent cause. They simply thought he was incredibly accident prone. Oddly, John became hypersensitive to certain aromas, like tea, which made him gag and vomit. He also experienced frequent ear infections and suffered permanent hearing loss.

The baby of the family, Phil, 3, was apparently not affected as badly as his older siblings. He did complain, however, of pain in his chest (sternum) and intermittent leg pains but no other significant symptoms.

After listening to Michelle relate each child's medical history as it might pertain to Lyme disease, the pediatrician asked her to bring them in for an evaluation. She did, and all the children were tested for Lyme disease. Michelle noted, "They all tested positive for Lyme from the beginning..."

As Michelle thought back on her children's diagnoses, she had to shake her head in disgust at what their former family pediatrician had said a couple of years before. Michelle recalled, "The pediatrician here in Boston said [my children] could not have Lyme disease because you cannot pass it along during pregnancy." Although environmental exposure is often difficult to rule out, the doctor's statement about fetal acquisition of the disease is contrary to published documentation. The O'Leary children certainly supported the documented observation of transplacental transfer of Borrelia burgdorferi from mother to fetus. Considering the ages of her three children and their unique symptoms, Michelle had sound reason to hope for a complete recovery for them.

Family in Treatment

Five months into Michelle's IV therapy, her children began their oral antibiotic treatments. Michelle's new resident nanny, *Nikki*, had her hands full assisting the family through what became a very difficult recovery. Michelle recalled, "We were all sick at the same time. We were all having terrible Herxheimer-like reactions and doing our best to keep diarrhea from the antibiotics in check. I would have to say, it was the most difficult time in all of our eyes."

The children's symptom flare-ups abated about three months into their treatments. Michelle was thankful for this because her own treatment period was far more difficult, and she could never have taken care of herself or the children without Nikki's help. She said, "I just continued with the worst Herxheimer-like reactions and ended up with Lyme meningitis twice in the first eight months of IV antibiotics along with a C. difficile infection in the intestines which required a month of Flagyl to treat it."

Michelle was spending a lot of time in bed during the initial period of her treatment. The children were off to school, and the house was so quiet. However, after school the children came up to Michelle's bedroom to visit on the bed with her for a little while. "They were such great company for me. We would read books or watch TV as we snuggled in bed," she remembered. Michelle was so thankful for

Nikki's help during that time. She managed the home and children for five years, and it made all the difference.

The children finished their oral antibiotic treatments after nine months, and Michelle was pleased with the outcomes. "John and Phil had no residual effects from Lyme disease although John did have some hearing loss. He [still] has to sit in the front of the class to hear properly. Phil is absolutely fine! Taylor [continues to] struggle with the neuropsychiatric manifestations of Lyme disease," Michelle explained.

Four years later, however, Taylor had to return to the doctor because she started to experience bad headaches and extreme photosensitivity. Obviously, her battle was not over, but she had a knowledgeable pediatrician and hope.

Long Island

During the summer of 2001, Michelle went through various trials and obstacles to recovery. First, her treating clinician moved away, so she had to find a new practitioner to continue her treatment. However, after she located a physician, he stopped her IV therapy and suggested she take oral antibiotics. Over the next three months, she tried five different oral antibiotics—none of them relieved her symptoms.

She knew she had to go back on IV therapy, but the doctor was afraid to risk his medical license to treat her in this manner. He said, "People are losing their licenses for treating patients such as you with long-term IV antibiotics. I, for one, cannot afford to lose my license. I am just starting out in my medical practice, and I have a lot of loans to pay off. I'm sorry."

Respecting his position on the issue, Michelle decided to keep looking for a doctor who would treat her long-term. In the process of her search, she began to realize that very few doctors were willing to treat Lyme disease beyond the standard guidelines of 4-6 weeks. This fact made her angry—not at the doctors—but at a system that censures and punishes physicians for trying to use extended antibiotic therapies to bring a patient to a symptom-free state of health. Now, in the middle of this medical debate, she had to find a doctor who would be willing to treat her despite the politics.

Then Michelle heard about a physician on the eastern end of Long Island, who used open-ended IV antibiotic therapy. She immediately made an appointment. Michelle anticipated the driving time involved—4½ hours one way—and she knew she would have to break up the trip into two days. She planned an overnight stay following her appointment, since Kevin was unable to take the time off from work to assist in the long commute. In any case, she felt the extra effort was worth it to check out this specialist.

At her appointment, the doctor reviewed her medical file—now five inches thick—and decided that she should return to IV therapy immediately. He prescribed Rocephin (ceftriaxone) because, he said, this drug could pass through the blood-brain barrier and be maintained at a level high enough to more effectively kill Lyme bacteria in the central nervous system.

Michelle agreed to the treatment protocol and remained on this therapy for about four months when her liver panel became elevated, indicating liver dysfunction. At this point, the doctor changed her prescription to Claforan. She successfully stayed on this medication for 1½ years, and during that time, her flare-up reactions gradually lessened in severity and frequency. This gave her reason to hope that one day, she would enjoy good health again. However, she still had occasional bouts of meningitis, and Michelle noted that recovery from these episodes took longer to achieve each time.

Her Happy Place

By late 2004, Michelle had regained about 60% of her former good health. "The incredible fatigue, muscle and bone pain are much improved, though I still need to take a nap every afternoon. My sleeping is slightly better, and the leg twitches and spasms are better controlled with Mirapex and Neurontin," she explained. The residual symptoms that still bother her include occasional depression (treated with Lexapro), leg weakness, bowel and bladder incontinence, severe headaches, occasional episodes of meningitis, left eye pain, and numbness and tingling along her right side.

For these residual symptoms, she continues to travel for monthly appointments to see her doctor on Long Island. On her return trips home, she sometimes visits the beach where she thinks about the direction her life has taken since 1990. She also ponders her losses—about the Camelot she once shared with Kevin and how her ill health has taken its toll on their marriage. "We have been in counseling now for close to three years. We both mourn the loss of our former selves," she said quietly as she stared out over the churning waves.

Michelle remembers herself as the "energetic, hard charger...with a plan. Kevin [was] the one willing to take the plan and go full steam ahead." Sadly, their once healthy and animated communication diminished to its present emaciated state—infrequent and lacking warmth. They are what Michelle calls "crimeless victims" in life. Frustration looms every time she thinks about the unnecessary obstacles she and Kevin faced in their search for a correct diagnosis and treatment of her illness. *It should not have been that way,* she thought. "My family and I have learned this lesson the hard way and paid the ultimate price of a healthy life together," she said.

All things considered, Michelle acknowledged that

there was no "her fault or his fault" in this tragic story. Life just happens—like the ocean, one never knows what will be washed up on shore the next day. By the same token, one never knows what the lapping waves will reclaim from those shores either. Life is as changeable and unpredictable as the ocean she finds so intriguingly consoling and mesmerizing. Perhaps there is a tragic irony in all of this, but she also knows that change can bring hope; and as a nurse, she knows how important hope is when battling a serious illness such as Lyme disease.

Facing Reality

Realistically, Michelle understood that some of the damage done to her body might be permanent. "I will never be able to run again, get through a day without a nap, or work in the profession I so loved. Instead, I have found other avenues to help me feel like a vital contributor to my family and society," she said. Suddenly, her father's words came to mind, "Those that can, do; those that can't, cheer for those that can." There was a time when Michelle was one of those "doers." Now she has learned to "cheer for those that can"—to help other Lyme patients avoid going through what she and her family had suffered. She found a new role in life, where her experience and skills as a nurse, patient, and seasoned medical consumer would have a positive impact.

Michelle now volunteers on the Tick-borne Disease Advisory Committee of the Massachusetts Department of Public Health and as a resource for information for the local Lyme disease support system. As a registered nurse, who had suffered greatly from chronic Lyme disease, Michelle speaks with hard-earned credentials as she gives public lectures on the disease. She also approaches schools to give teachers and school nurses information on a disease that affects thousands of children each year. After all, Lyme disease, along with other tick-borne illnesses, are among the fastest growing infectious diseases in America, and if not caught early and left untreated, disability and personal tragedy may occur.

Michelle keeps an open mind toward all new treatments that might alleviate her remaining Lyme disease and co-infection symptoms. Around Thanksgiving of 2004, she was treated with an intravenous immunoglobulin (IVIg) called gamma globulin. Intravenous gamma globulin is made from pooled human blood that is washed and processed until it is clear in appearance. The resulting sterile protein that remains from this process is then transfused into the patient. This is considered an experimental approach for treating Lyme disease. Michelle said, "It helps some people, but it didn't help me. I reacted adversely to the treatment with aseptic meningitis twice and had to be hospitalized for a few days each time." After the last treatment in early January 2005, Michelle said, "I am having terrible problems with my vision. There was something going on causing a horrible headache and left eye pain." As a result, any further plans to treat Michelle with IVIg were abandoned.

Once again, she was placed on IV antibiotics, but by early March, she was admitted to the hospital with sepsis from her third port. "They removed the port, and then I was discharged home on oral antibiotics to treat the Lyme," she said. Michelle admitted that she never had any success with oral antibiotics, so she did not hold out any hope for good results from her latest prescription.

Further discouragement followed when, on two different occasions during the ensuing months, Michelle underwent an MRI of her spinal cord. The news was not good either time—the images showed an increased number of lesions in the thoracic spinal cord area. Still, Michelle continued her antibiotic therapy, and in early December, she was admitted to the hospital for a few days to be treated for a leg condition diagnosed as spasticity, which is also common in MS patients.

Clearly, since Michelle's correct diagnosis, her life has been consumed fighting chronic Lyme disease. She has won some battles and lost others, but the fight wages on. One thing is certain, she cannot afford to drop her vigilance or her determination to fight, because each day promises change and new hope. Michelle's love for her family motivates her to keep seeking answers to this complex illness. As a medical professional and researcher, she knows that one day, a new treatment may be discovered that will work in her case.

Final Reflections

The medical history of Michelle O'Leary demonstrates how illness can cause a complete reversal of one's circumstances. Camelot had been stolen from the O'Leary couple shortly after their marriage. Now it is just a brief memory for Michelle and Kevin. They know, all too well, that serious illness will test the strength of a marriage and the unity of the family—either it will pull together, become divided, or in some other way show dysfunction. However, with love and understanding, a family can survive serious illness.

That is why Michelle's forewarning strongly addresses families. "You absolutely have to have the support of your spouse for two reasons," she said, "One—to support you and be an advocate with these physicians. Two—if you have children, your spouse needs to reassure them that you will be okay." She learned that illness affects everyone in the home, and it must be approached as a family if the family intends to survive intact.

Furthermore, she advises patients never to give up— not even when physicians and family members don't believe you. Michelle set the right example and stayed the course. She listened intuitively to her own body and did her own medical research. "No one had more at stake in finding the proper diagnosis than me," she said.

Though Michelle was misdiagnosed for 10 years, she persevered. She saw numerous specialists, went to well known clinics, and availed herself of some of the best medical resources available. When she refused to believe their nebulous diagnoses, she was told to "stop being a wimp" or "tough it out." She was asked to "give up" on these silly notions that she had Lyme disease. Even among Lyme disease "specialists," she found great variance in expertise, knowledge, and opinion. Not surprisingly then, Michelle advises patients "[You] are the one paying the doctors' salaries and [so] never take any diagnosis or treatment with blind faith."

As a former member of the medical system, Michelle discovered some irony in being a nurse-patient. On one hand, it offered some advantages for her as a patient, but also some unexpected disadvantages. "I know being a nurse many times was a hindrance as people assumed [I] knew everything, and [so I] got few explanations. I also found that nurses are intimidated by nurses as patients, which resulted in a few medical mishaps," she said.

Despite these past experiences, Michelle intends to stay focused on her treatment options in hopes of eliminating her remaining symptoms. She also awaits the introduction of new antibiotics which may hold promise for greater improvement. Medicine is ever-evolving, and this fact alone offers reason for chronic Lyme patients to persevere.

Whatever the future brings, she has learned that there is always hope. "I am not [an] overly religious [person], but [I] do believe that when God closes a door, He opens a window," she said. Michelle is hoping that when she looks through that window, she will, once again, have a panoramic view of Camelot.

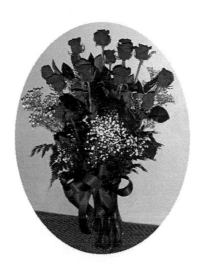

The Love of My Life

"...we have much more to fear from the
deficiency of truth, than from its abundance."
—*Caleb C. Colton*

Anyone who has lost the greatest love of their
life knows the depth of pain that follows,
said *Rhonda* as her sullen eyes dropped
to her lap where she caressed her yellow tabby. Life had
changed dramatically for her since December 1, 2003, when
her husband, *George*, 58, died from neuroborreliosis—a
nervous system infection by Borrelia burgdorferi. "It hasn't
been easy," she added. After his death, she had to sell their
cottage to pay the bills, and today, she lives in a mobile home
park in a small community in New Jersey. Her life is much
more quiet these days—plenty of time to sort through 12
years of memories shared with George.

He had a very privileged childhood with opportunities

that few get to enjoy. "George had an exceptionally active and demanding childhood and adolescence. He was a model and an actor. He did many different ads for various products. [He was involved with] Broadway and off Broadway plays and summer stock," Rhonda said. During his years of association with the theater and movies, he saw plenty of backstage action, but none interested him more than the duties of the stage electricians.

His curiosity developed into experimentation, and eventually, he became very proficient at performing electrical tasks. In his early adulthood, he attended school and became a licensed electrician. He became gainfully employed at a union job in a well known theme park. In his spare time, he also worked as an electrician in his own business. He took his occupation very seriously because lives depended upon his knowledge and expertise—especially at the theme park—where thousands of people trusted the mechanical and electrical integrity of the high speed, thrill rides.

Aside from his job, George's personal life centered around home, his personal electrical business, and his social circle of church friends. He was a well liked man with a lot of friends. Known for his empathy and nonjudgmental disposition, George was often the person others sought when they needed a listening ear or a word of comfort. He was generous with his time, and he genuinely cared about others.

Rhonda, who owned and operated a floral shop in town, had known George since the early 1980s. She watched him go through two marriages before life brought them together in 1997. They enjoyed their courtship—going out for dinner, taking in a movie at the theater, or watching a foreign film at home. Their companionship was exciting and felt very natural. On warm, summer weekends, George uncovered his 1983 911SC Porsche and took Rhonda on long drives—often with no particular destination in mind. Sometimes they got lost in the process, but they were unconcerned as long as they were together. Other times, they drove into the city simply to talk over a steamy cup of cappuccino. It was the best of times as this middle-aged couple discovered new love—fresh, romantic, and unconditional.

Troubling Symptoms

During this same period of time, George began to notice that his attention span seemed short-circuited and that he felt uncommon mood swings. For a man who was usually very amicable, the mood swings seemed very abnormal, and this concerned him to the point where he consulted a psychiatrist. After evaluation, the psychiatrist diagnosed George with adult attention deficit disorder (ADD) and treated him with an ongoing prescription of Ritalin. Shortly after seeing the psychiatrist, he also began to experience increased instances of memory recall dysfunction. Thinking that this might somehow be associated with ADD, he didn't see the doctor for this symptom. However, not long afterward, he also began feeling unusually fatigued during the day. He struggled with frequent bouts of depression, which he had never experienced to this degree before. More alarming than this, George began to suffer from recurring bouts of pneumonia, which occurred about every other month. His doctor put him on antibiotics, and he would improve, but he invariably relapsed shortly after finishing his course of medication.

Finally by March 1999, George felt he could no longer keep working under such circumstances. With his concentration difficulties, he felt he could not guarantee the integrity of his work at the theme park. His fatigue, depression, and time away from work to recover from pneumonia was taking its toll on him. Consequently, he consulted his doctor who validated George's request to leave work on temporary disability. Interestingly, during this consultation, the doctor tested George for Lyme disease, and an ELISA (antibody test) was performed, but the results were negative.

What began as a temporary disability in March 1999, developed into a prolonged leave of absence as George's symptoms persisted and worsened. His employer agreed that it was in everyone's best interest that George take whatever time off he needed to recover before returning to his job. After all, competent theme park maintenance was critical to safety, and lives depended on the quality of the maintenance work performed. If George suffered from frequent forgetfulness or was in any way distracted from the vital details of his work, the personal injury and liability issues simply could not allow him to continue. George understood all of that, and he wanted nothing better than to recover. Unfortunately, no one knew exactly what was wrong with him.

An Alarming Diagnosis

On June 6, 1999, George was admitted to the emergency room (ER) at the local medical center. This was, in fact, the second time he had been admitted to the emergency room within a week. George was very ill this time. His speech was stuttering and incoherent, and he seemed confused and extremely weak.

While George was being examined, the attending ER physician told George that he should be admitted into the hospital for testing by other specialists. George consented, and after several tests were performed, the results were not at all what they expected to hear. Rhonda explained, "The doctor told me that George had incurable and inoperable lung cancer that spread to his brain. He told me there was nothing he could do but keep him out of pain by using a morphine drip." George bowed his head and cried—to think that his life would end in this way and so soon. The brevity of life, the injustice of premature death—these thoughts came flooding into his heart and mind with enormous emotional force.

No one could have foretold this moment. Admittedly, Rhonda recognized that George had lost considerable weight during the past year and that he was extremely fatigued, but she never thought he had cancer! She looked at George resting in his hospital bed and could not believe how quickly his health had deteriorated. As far as George's physician was concerned, the hospital was going to be his last place of residence before his death. It was a depressing thought.

Rhonda tried to balance her time between hospital visits and operating her floral shop. Somehow she was able to do it all, but each time she visited George's hospital room, she noticed its constant, deplorable condition. The room smelled of urine so strongly that Rhonda decided to scrub the floor herself. Despite using strong detergents and scrubbing on her hands and knees, the smell persisted. She ultimately realized that the urine smell was emanating from the walls, and there was virtually nothing that could be done about it.

As for George's care, Rhonda was alarmed at the hospital staff's obvious patient neglect. She said, "His food tray was put down in front of him, and not once did I see anyone assist him to eat." Rhonda fed him and also dealt with his occasional violent displays of dementia. However, despite her attention and caregiving, he gradually became unresponsive. "He was [like] a vegetable—could not talk, walk, stand, lift his arms—nothing at all," said Rhonda. The only way he was able to communicate with her was by squeezing her hand once for "yes" and twice for "no." It was heart wrenching to see the love of her life, a 54-year-old, intelligent electrician, slip away so quickly.

After 16 days, George was discharged from the hospital and transferred to a rehabilitation center where physical therapists worked with him to improve his large motor skills and speech. Rhonda was pleased with the attention he received there, but she was even more pleased at what the doctors at the center concluded from additional diagnostic testing. "After many tests...the doctors there were not able to diagnose him, but [they] did rule out lung cancer and brain cancer. I was just grateful at this time that the [hospital] doctors were wrong," Rhonda said.

After the good news, Rhonda and George were informed that there was one minor health condition that the tests did reveal, and that this condition was treatable. Apparently, George had a small pocket of clear fluid on one lung. This was successfully siphoned out, and the rest of his lung tissue appeared clear, pink, and healthy.

Home Healthcare

George had been in the rehabilitation center for 56 days when his doctor approached Rhonda and told her that he was not progressing with this therapy at the rate he had hoped. That being the case, he wanted to transfer George to a subacute facility where he could continue his therapy on his own. With a little investigating, Rhonda realized that such a facility was nothing more than a nursing home with an exercise room. A referral to a facility like this was not an acceptable option for George. What he needed was continued one-on-one physical therapy sessions, so Rhonda immediately contacted their insurance company's case worker who suggested an alternative plan.

Rhonda explained, "I arranged for George to return home [and receive] physical, speech, and cognitive therapy on location at home." She had hired carpenters to make the house handicap friendly prior to his discharge, and then she approached the physician with her idea. The doctor at the rehabilitation center agreed, and on August 17, 1999, George was discharged home.

George was very excited to return home after being away for 72 days. As Rhonda pushed him in his wheelchair into the house, he said, "Oh, I'm so glad to be back." His cat, Gizmo, quickly jumped onto his lap to greet him. George was all smiles and so thrilled to receive such a welcome from his old pal. Rhonda immediately showed him all the remodeling that she ordered done in the house for his convenience. As a finale, she took him outside again to the garage and uncovered his "girl," his Porsche. She started the engine for him and let it run for a while because he always loved the sound of his baby's engine.

George's positive reaction to his home surroundings affirmed that home was exactly where he needed to be. He could have been transferred to another nursing home, but they wanted to prevent what they called "doctor hopping." Every time George changed healthcare facilities, he was assigned to a new doctor, and the cycle of re-evaluations began all over again. George and Rhonda felt this just consumed precious time, and they wanted to avoid that if at all possible. Since George really liked the neurologist he met at the rehabilitation center, he wanted to continue his patient-doctor relationship with him until he recovered.

Philadelphia Doctor

In September 1999, Rhonda and George had their first consultation with the neurologist since his discharge from the rehabilitation center. He examined George and reread his medical history to date. Rhonda said, "He told [us] that George was a mystery to him and [to] all the doctors at the rehabilitation [center]." The neurologist said he could prescribe something for George's tremors, but he did not feel qualified or experienced enough to give him a proper diagnosis.

Having said that, he recommended a referral to a

specialist and colleague with whom he had worked while at a hospital in Philadelphia. He felt certain that this physician would be able to help George. An appointment was scheduled for October 18, and George left the neurologist's office hoping this wasn't going to be the beginning of the doctor hopping that he wanted to avoid.

At this consultation, George was examined and diagnosed with a rare brain stem multiple sclerosis (MS). The doctor subsequently prescribed a fairly new, injectable drug called Avonex (an interferon with very strong adverse effects). Rhonda was taught how to administer this drug intramuscularly (IM) once a week. He was also given other treatments, the combination of which produced very frightening results.

"The most aggressive treatment ordered was Cytoxin chemotherapy and Solu-Medrol [cortico]steroid infusions, once a month for six months," Rhonda said. George started on this regimen in November, and it appeared, at first, that he was tolerating the chemotherapy well and that the corticosteroid medication was giving him strength. However, his treatment was interrupted for one month while he took antibiotics to treat a case of pneumonia. After he recovered from that, chemotherapy resumed.

Amidst all the doctor appointments and treatments, George and Rhonda realized they shared a mature love for one another, and they declared their commitment with marriage vows in April 2000. It was a moment of time that was as peaceful as anyone could imagine. The wedding took place in a neighbor's back yard. The yard itself was manicured and decorated like something out of a *Better Homes and Gardens* magazine. Seating was arranged for their 25 guests, and the wedding took place at noon under a gorgeous, blue sky. The mayor, a long time friend, officiated over the wedding, and friends shared in their joy at the cake cutting and Italian buffet following the ceremony.

George's illness did not overshadow their wedding day. It was stimulating to him to be surrounded by friends who shared the joy of that day with him. He and Rhonda enjoyed opening gifts together in front of their friends, but as evening approached, George began to show signs of exhaustion from a joyous but overwhelming day. It was a reminder to them both that their trials were still present. However, they also were comforted by the thought that they would face the unknown future together.

In June, while George was still on his aggressive therapy, he became extremely weak and sick. As a result, the doctor ordered another MRI. He wanted to compare the current images to those taken in November 1999. What he saw was remarkable. Rhonda said, "The MS lesions were no longer active, and the white and gray matter was starting to [heal] too." Consequently, the doctor took George off the corticosteroid medication and chemotherapy protocol in order to give his body a rest.

IV Antibiotic Therapy

Unfortunately, he did not feel rested at all. By that August, he had become very ill, and Rhonda took him to be examined by their primary care physician. Tests were performed, and an abscess was located on George's lung. He was immediately admitted to the hospital where more tests were conducted over the next week. Finally, the doctor ordered the installation of a Hickman catheter and a six week course of IV antibiotics that George would take at home.

In addition to his therapy, George received visits from home healthcare providers and the services of an excellent cognitive therapist. Over the next nine months, he responded well to therapy, and he showed progressive physical and cognitive improvement. "The infection cleared, and he seemed to be doing a lot better. He was showering and dressing on his own. [He] had full control of his bladder and bowels and was able to read and write a little," Rhonda recalled. It seemed like George had undergone a miraculous transformation—from being an unresponsive patient to one who was ambulatory with recuperating cognitive abilities.

Despite the fact that he had made such marked improvement, George was very frustrated that he had lost his fluent speech. For someone whose words were once so healing to others, he now had trouble selecting simple words to express himself. "I hate this!" he told Rhonda in utter frustration. He couldn't help but compare himself to the man he used to be. His home was filled with reminders of this— his wall photos, his personal belongings, and his Porsche parked in the garage—they all spoke of past activities and pursuits in life that he loved. Clearly, his quality of life had diminished, and this fact contributed to further depression.

On June 28, 2001, George was admitted to the hospital for what was later diagnosed as a relapse of MS. Again, he was placed on high doses of Solu-Medrol corticosteroids. This had a detrimental effect upon George as Rhonda explained. "He went into [cortico]steroid psychosis and never fully recovered from that." Another MRI was performed, and it showed no changes from the previous images taken in June 2000. The doctor was very puzzled over what was causing George's extreme fatigue and cognitive dysfunction.

Over the next few months, George grew weaker, and the relatively healthy spans between treatments became shorter over time. In the past, he used to leave home for physical therapy sessions, but now, severe fatigue made that impossible, so in-home therapy was arranged.

A Florida Vacation

Due to the cost of George's medical care, he and Rhonda were forced to sell their home and move into their cottage. Following the move, they decided to take a modest trip to Florida—the first vacation they had taken since 1997 and a badly needed distraction from George's health issues. They were in Florida to ring in the 2002 New Year, but after that, their holiday took a downturn. George complained to Rhonda, "I don't feel well. I feel like I'm going to have a heart attack, and I can't breathe right." Rhonda did the only thing she could do under the circumstances—she called 911 for an ambulance. She followed the ambulance in her car and accompanied George as he was admitted to the local hospital. She hadn't thought to bring any of his medical records with them on vacation, but she did her best to relate his complicated medical history to the attending neurologist.

After listening to Rhonda and examining George for his presenting complaints, the doctor ordered another MRI. After examining the images, the discerning neurologist told Rhonda, "Something was eating his brain, and [I] don't think it is MS." This came as a real surprise to Rhonda and George. Rhonda told the doctor that a knowledgeable neurologist in Philadelphia had diagnosed George with MS. The Florida doctor was not impressed and responded frankly, "That means nothing." He was the first medical professional to suggest that something other than MS might be the cause of George's condition, and Rhonda was determined to pursue this topic with the Philadelphia neurologist as soon as they returned home.

When that appointment arrived, the neurologist looked at the Florida films and compared them to earlier ones. Almost apologetically, the doctor told George and Rhonda that there were no remarkable changes in the new images. The physician had nothing more to say because he saw no medical evidence to change his previous diagnosis of MS. The couple left his office, disappointed and somewhat confused over the difference of professional opinion concerning his MS diagnosis.

Symptoms Worsen

The following month of February 2002 brought worsening symptoms for George. He suffered with severe depression and experienced daylong crying spells. At his psychologist's advice, he admitted himself into a psychiatric ward at the hospital for care, but he received no relief from his psychosis. Rhonda said, "That was a complete waste of time. They were of no help at all."

George was discharged only to be readmitted in early March to the local hospital. His doctor ordered another MRI, and after examining the images, he stated that he thought George was experiencing a relapse of MS. Again, the doctor prescribed a treatment involving high doses of corticosteroids, but this time they had no strengthening effect on George. Even the physical therapist reported that George was not responding to therapy as well as he had in the past. The therapist explained that unless he acquired greater strength, he would not qualify for outpatient physical therapy services.

Rhonda immediately called to make an appointment for George with the doctor in Philadelphia, but the earliest available opening was in May. Rhonda accepted that date, but over the next few days, she noted, "George was so sick by [the second week in March], that I thought he would die before May." In a desperate attempt to receive help from this physician, Rhonda and George drove to Philadelphia to his office on March 10, 2002. They arrived almost two months in advance of his appointment—unannounced—and they waited in the office lobby until the doctor had time to see George.

The doctor compared the MRIs from the hospital in Florida to those taken during George's early March admission to their local hospital. After taking a deep sigh, he told them the dire news—it appeared as though the lesions were active and spreading. The doctor prescribed an aggressive treatment of Novantrone, which is highly destructive to rapidly proliferating cells in all stages of cell division. It is frequently used to treat some cancers and progressive relapses of multiple sclerosis. The drug can increase the risk of infections.

George returned home to begin his new treatment. However, on April 17, he was again admitted to the hospital in Pennsylvania where he was submitted to corticosteroid therapy again. This time, the treatment did not even offer him a false sense of energy, as it had at times in the past. Due to his severe fatigue, it was impossible for him to commute back and forth to his outpatient physical therapy sessions. His circumstances, medicines, and his mysterious illness contributed toward deep depression.

His psychosis, this time, was more severe than ever before. Rhonda explained, "He had horrible crying spells, hallucinations, and unbearable fear. He repeated everything that I would say. He was thinking we were in strange places when we were at home. I felt so bad for him and so helpless." The physician in Pennsylvania recommended that George resume his Novantrone treatment, and he went back on this harsh drug in May. Home healthcare services were ordered which allowed George to have in-home physical therapy again.

An Amazing Discovery

By June, Rhonda and George had learned how MS and Lyme disease can present with very similar symptoms. It was only when they began to talk about Lyme disease that George recalled, "I had been bitten by a tick in 1987 at work." He went on to relate that a rash appeared behind his knee on one of his calves, and he showed it to the company nurse. She looked at it, but apparently did not recognize it as an erythema migrans rash associated with Lyme disease. Instead, she cautioned him to watch it and to seek treatment if he experienced troubling symptoms. Since the rash disappeared shortly thereafter, George gave it no further thought until now.

Rhonda immediately located a doctor in the area who was familiar with treating Lyme disease, and she made an appointment for George. During his first, thorough, clinical evaluation, blood was drawn to run Western blot tests for Lyme disease. At their next meeting in mid-July, the doctor told George that he tested positive on one Western blot. His first reaction was one of surprise and then disgust. He said, "For three years, I had been betrayed by the medical community into thinking I had MS when I didn't." Now that there was medical evidence of Lyme disease, he only hoped that he had been diagnosed in time to be successfully treated.

The doctor recommended a treatment protocol involving IV Rocephin for at least two to three months. The treatment was scheduled to begin as soon as Rhonda could arrange for the necessary in-home healthcare services. Until then, the doctor prescribed oral antibiotics for George to take at home. The physician cautioned that in his situation, the illness would be difficult to treat since so many immunosuppressant drugs had been used, and the disease would be very fully entrenched in George's system. Despite this, George was hopeful that he would improve and so grateful that he had a strong advocate in Rhonda.

Shortly after he began taking oral antibiotics, George noticed that his ankles were swollen and that the swelling was traveling downward into his feet. "George's feet looked twice their normal size. He was complaining about his head and [that he] couldn't move," Rhonda said. She became alarmed and called 911 for an ambulance. She followed

George to the hospital and brought his Western blot results along to share with the attending physician.

The neurologist at the hospital studied the test results and the notes from the Lyme disease doctor outlining her recommended treatment for George. Since he was still taking oral antibiotics, the neurologist immediately ordered the administration of IV Rocephin to more aggressively attack the disease. At 10:00 p.m. on the evening of July 20, 2002, George received his first dose of IV Rocephin. He was in a weakened state at this time, so the doctor transferred him to the subacute floor of the hospital where he was given physical therapy to help strengthen him. Disappointed, Rhonda said, "It didn't really stabilize him. The [staff] made errors with his medications, too."

Throughout this terrible ordeal, Rhonda learned how essential it was to become a medical advocate for her sick loved one. At the hospital where George had been a patient, she observed all levels of professional competence and incompetence. Some patient care practices were alarmingly deficient, and she learned from hard experience that it was imperative to remain a vigilant advocate for George—be his eyes and ears especially after his illness progressed neurologically and cognitively.

A Guarded Prognosis

After a short time in subacute care, George was discharged home. He continued under the care of two physicians, the Lyme disease doctor and the neurologist who had recently treated George at the hospital. His condition was grave, and he showed little improvement. Rhonda said, "George had lost most of his mental capability and [frequently] pulled out his IV's. He was getting worse each month." His physicians told Rhonda that because George's case of Lyme disease was diagnosed late—years late—and that he had been on harsh immunosuppressants for an extended time period, no promising medical prognosis could be made.

Rhonda was attentive to George at home. He loved her home cooked meals and her company. "We were a team. We wouldn't give up trying," Rhonda recalled. After nearly a year on IV antibiotics, his symptoms lessened and stabilized. Though he was still in a wheelchair, he had periods of greater alertness followed by several days in bed. This was definitely an improvement for George. Finally, in June 2003, he finished his IV antibiotic therapy.

However, one month later, new and troubling symptoms appeared. George developed a constant cough and was having difficulty swallowing. He saw an ear, nose, and throat (ENT) specialist several times over the course of the next two months. Finally, the ENT ordered a diagnostic procedure called a barium swallow. With difficulty, George submitted to the test, and the results confirmed what they had already known—that George was unable to swallow properly. Based on these results, the doctor recommended that a feeding tube be inserted into George's stomach.

This was not exactly good news to George, whose last luxury was Rhonda's good cooking. However, on September 26, George was admitted to the hospital and the procedure was performed without difficulty. He stayed in the hospital for about a week, during which time, George was put back on an IV antibiotic. Rhonda feared it was too late, though. She said, "He was in rough shape. [He had] one more short round of home physical therapy and health aids. I knew in my heart that I was now beginning to lose him for sure." With somber acceptance, Rhonda decided she would make his time left as comfortable as she possibly could.

Hospice Care

Rhonda transformed a room in their cottage into a hospital room for George. A hospital bed was brought in, and Rhonda helped George in and out of it several times each day to give him a change of posture and scenery. This was very difficult at times because George felt so dizzy that he struggled with Rhonda in the process of being transferred. It was at this point in time, that the home health nurses suggested that Rhonda ask his doctor to order Hospice care. However, George was so afraid of dying that Rhonda thought the presence of Hospice care in their home would be too much for him.

Putting this decision off for a while longer, Rhonda started to read books to him during his wakeful periods. He particularly enjoyed listening to stories of a spiritual nature and stories about others like him, who were facing imminent death. He found strength in their stories, and he wanted to prepare himself. A close friend of Rhonda's came over to pray with and for him. He was very grateful for this comfort and support and said, "I'm glad I have God."

The Last Act of Love

The week following Thanksgiving 2003 was extremely difficult for George. He labored for each breath. Rhonda asked the home health nurse if she ought to call Hospice at that time, but the nurse suggested waiting until the following Monday. That Monday morning, George was so ill that Rhonda called an ambulance. She recalled, "It was the first time I rode in the ambulance with him. I used to always follow in my car, but I wanted to be with him at his side to comfort him." As they sped away from their home to the hospital, she knew this was his last trip to the hospital and that he would not be coming home again.

When they arrived at the emergency room, the attending physician diagnosed him with a severe case of pneumonia as a complication of MS. He advised her that "it didn't look like it would be long." Rhonda's mind went blank, shocked for a moment by the rawness of those unwelcome words and the knowledge that their time together was slipping away. She quickly returned to George's bedside to comfort him. She took his hand and prayed just loud enough for him to hear. Bending toward him, she whispered her last goodbye into his ear, and then he was gone.

The realities of his death were slow to absorb and slower to accept. Rhonda lingered by George's still body, unwilling to leave him and in disbelief that he was no longer breathing. Finally, her sister arrived to take her home. Home—how quiet it seemed now. The hospital bed was there, but the love of her life was gone. There was no longer any need for Rhonda's caregiving—her job was finished. That fateful morning of December 1, 2003, had changed everything that was familiar and loved in her life, and she felt a profound sense of loss and of being lost.

The next month was spent doing the solemn paperwork that death produces. In the process, she examined his death certificate and noticed that his cause of death was recorded as "end stages of multiple sclerosis." Rhonda knew differently, and she wanted the record to correctly include Lyme disease as the underlying cause of his MS-like symptoms. Therefore, Rhonda acquired the Lyme disease doctor's diagnosis and had George's death certificate officially corrected to state the cause of his death as "the end stage of multiple sclerosis *as a consequence of neuroborreliosis (infection of the nervous system by Borrelia burgdorferi)."*

More than a year later, Rhonda said of her experience, "Anyone who has lost the greatest love of their life knows the rest. It isn't easy." Although she is comforted in knowing that George's suffering came to an end, she hopes and prays that his illness may serve as a warning to others. She wants it known that Lyme disease can be fatal when left untreated or treated with drugs that compromise the immune system, and George's experience demonstrated that sad fact.

Few case reports of death due to complications from Lyme disease can be found in the scientific literature. The currently accepted conclusion is that fatal outcomes from this disease are rare and are usually an indirect result of the disease process. While death may be infrequent, actually defining "rare" in terms of statistics can only occur if unbiased and thorough analyses are undertaken. Such evaluations should also include deaths due to suicide and the contribution of co-infections to any fatal outcomes.

Rhonda advised that if anyone suspects they have contracted Lyme disease, get diagnosed and treated early. "Run—don't walk—to a doctor that specializes in Lyme disease. Call your local Lyme disease association and get a referral [because] Lyme disease kills," she said with a tone of finality.

Incidentally, in October 2002, while caring for George, Rhonda was also diagnosed with Lyme disease. She suffers from debilitating symptoms and is currently undergoing treatment.

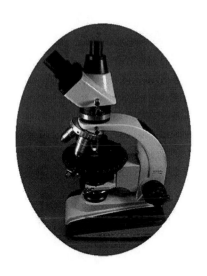

A Scientist's Dilemma

"Life is short; death is long."
—*Edwin Lilley Sr.*

Somewhere between theory and practical wisdom lies the battlefield of truth where science and medicine attempt to understand and explain the mysteries of microbiology. At times, however, science and medicine appear at odds with each other. It was precisely this type of situation that created a critical and personal dilemma for environmental health specialist, *Edwin Lilley,* of Seattle.

When he experienced the onset of a rapidly degenerative illness, he sought to investigate its origin. He applied what he knew—science—and what he learned surprised him. The origin of his illness was not an obvious toxin, such as those he frequently encountered in his work among the solvents, acids, and heavy metal wastes of some

287

methamphetamine lab crime scene.   No—quite to the contrary—the search for his truth led him to a place he least expected.

"Who would think that one little tick hanging out in a campground in Provincetown, Massachusetts, would send me on the path to the road to ruin?   The evils that people normally look out for [here] are crystal meth, bad disco music, hangovers, and contracting AIDS—not Lyme disease—but that's what happened to me in 1996," he said.

Everything in his life has changed since then. What was once a life with seemingly endless possibilities has become one of ending possibilities—a sedentary shadow of the passionate, almost reckless life he once led. Though he has been dealing with the disabilities caused by his illness, memories of his former life before Lyme disease still give rise to understandable anger and mourning.

A Reckless Love

Born during the social revolution of the mid-1960s, Ed was raised and influenced by two talented and outrageously eccentric parents. His mother, an artist, and his father, a scientist, allowed Ed a great deal of latitude growing up in their home on Long Island's North Shore. Not surprisingly, then, he immersed himself in every whim and dream that inspired him. "I raced sailboats in the summer and went to prep school up north in Vermont in the winter. [My parents] nurtured my love of danger, but that did not preclude social responsibility." They reminded him, "The wages of sin will get you nowhere." No argument with God on that score, but in terms of immediate gratification and pleasure, Ed also believed that "sin could also be a whole lot of fun."

Thrill seeking, adventuresome, and a carefree globetrotter, Ed admitted he thought youth should be spent living life to its fullest. After all, "life is short; death is long," his father used to remind him. Little did he know, though, that the kind of explorative lifestyle he enjoyed might come at a long-term cost to him personally. "I had a reckless love of the outdoors, which made me a prime candidate for Lyme," Ed explained in hindsight.

He was athletic, healthy, and craved the thrills and dangers that the outdoors offered. "I sailed boats on Oyster Bay in hurricanes, climbed Mt. Washington in New Hampshire's White Mountains during a winter whiteout in 100-plus mile an hour winds. [I] bicycled through France during the summer at the age of 15; camped in farmers' fields and in Paris' notorious Bois de Boulogne, which [by day] was a gorgeous park, [but, at night] became an open air market for transvestite prostitutes."

Back in the States, Ed "bike toured through New England and rode the 350 mile trip from New York to boarding school in Vermont every fall, camping in the woods at night."

Working as a bike messenger in Manhattan provided him with a daily dose of adrenaline and thrills as he maneuvered his Peugeot racing bike through the crazy maze of cars and pedestrians on his way to various delivery destinations.

Hiking also offered all kinds of excitement for Ed. He trekked the Metacomet-Monadnock Trail through Massachusetts and New Hampshire, and he also hiked through the gorgeous Grand Canyon. Most of his travel to and from these areas was done by hitchhiking. This, too, was a thrilling sport to him. Meeting, talking, and traveling with strangers was part of the entire experience. "I hitchhiked all over the Northeast, living out of my backpack and tent," he said. All of these adventures, not to mention his love of downhill ski racing, were the order and substance of Ed's life—that is—before he turned 18 years old.

Education

In every sense of the word, Ed's world was his classroom; however, in terms of secondary educational institutions, he attended what he called "the socially progressive" Vershire School in Vermont. This boarding school suited Ed well because, as he admitted, "it had very few rules." It did, however, have a college level curriculum and a great environmental science program, which really appealed to him.

Though Ed never had to worry about financing his education, he did have some personal expenses that he had to assume on his own. "I worked to pay my expenses, raising pigs, tapping maple trees for sap, and doing other exciting things like fixing leaky sewage pipes on cold winter nights." For fun, he spent his school breaks following the rock band performances of The Grateful Dead. In the summer, he lived in Manhattan's East Village and explored the "vibrant art scene in those days." He witnessed artists, Jean Michel Basquiat and Keith Haring start their careers there. That was all sedate entertainment to Ed; whereas, attending punk rock shows "with friends and sneaking into The Mudd Club and The Pyramid Club with our fake I.D.'s," was a bit more stimulating for him.

That's how Ed spent his boarding school years. Time passed quickly, and he graduated. Before he knew it, his college years arrived. He ultimately enrolled in three different colleges—Marlboro College in Vermont, the Evergreen State College in Washington, and Franklin Pierce College in New Hampshire.

While attending college in New Hampshire, he lived in a wood heated cabin in the wilderness. It had barely any amenities to speak of—no running water—just an outhouse.

The more primitive, the more Ed enjoyed it. He embraced the rustic life, the isolation, and being able to surround himself with all that was natural. During the winters when the New Hampshire snows blanketed the ground, he brought out his cross country skis and traveled to and from classes this way. Reminiscing, he said, "It was a great life!"

While attending college, Ed also became involved in political activism—it was an education outside the forum of a classroom. "I protested the gentrification of developers kicking out the poor in New York; [I] sat on railroad tracks that carried radioactive materials destined for use in nuclear weapons; [I] learned about the power of civil disobedience." He also zealously participated in the 1988 Democratic presidential campaign and enjoyed the perks associated with that. In character, he said, "Michael Dukakis always had the best booze and food, but Jessie Jackson always had cold beer in the bathtub and a more fun crowd."

In the formal classrooms of college, Ed enrolled in many liberal arts courses, which he enjoyed thoroughly, but his career focus was in the environmental sciences. "I studied the policy side and natural science side of the environmental sciences, [but] I found that environmental science departments did a poor job of training future environmentalists about social policy and natural science issues." For this reason, Ed designed his own college major—Human Ecology—and in 1989, he graduated cum laude from Franklin Pierce College.

The Bureaucratic Treadmill

After graduation, Ed found work with The Nature Conservancy, conducting flowering plant surveys. Later, he was appointed to the conservation commission in the New Hampshire town where he lived, and he handled public health issues and environmental policy problems that emerged as a result of converting rural areas into housing developments. Eventually, Ed changed jobs and began work as a public health sanitarian for the city of Nashua, New Hampshire. In this public office, he conducted rat population surveys, monitored public drinking water supplies, and worked in the microbiology lab. It was, in all respects, the fulfillment of his career objectives.

Despite this, he was growing increasingly restless. At the close of each work day, he eagerly looked forward to the peaceful seclusion of his rustic cabin home in the woods. Even there, however, he found himself contemplating the next day's work tasks. He began to feel shackled to the bureaucratic system that employed him, and he resented it.

Having been born into some wealth, Ed felt he had a choice whether or not to work at this time in his life. In all honesty, he did not want to spend his young adulthood in servitude to public health. It was a turning point in his life and a wake up call of sorts. He thought, "Youth is wasted on the young," and he didn't want to waste anymore time on this bureaucratic treadmill—at least not right now. He had places to go and people to see, and time was ticking away.

Youthful Hiatus

Without a second thought, Ed quit his job and returned to Europe. There, he bought a Eurail pass and traveled extensively over the next year. The 100,000 mile rail network transported him throughout the European countries including England and Ireland. He traveled from Amsterdam to the beaches of Monaco's mythic Monte-Carlo and many places in-between. He hiked through the Swiss Alps and backpacked through Liechtenstein.

"[I] slept in my tent or crashed in hostels. I traveled to the still communist country of Hungary, where I bribed my way out of jail, went to an opera every night in Budapest,

[and] hit the underground clubs with friends, drinking beer in the ancient caverns below the city and nursing my hangovers at the hot spring spas the next day. I never lived so well," said Ed.

It was a backpacker's life, and he loved it. Eventually, though, he came back to the United States and found work again. "[I] ran a bookstore for the Antioch New England Graduate School." Knowing that Ed wanted to travel to the Pacific Northwest to live in Seattle, his friends threw a keg, fund raising party to pay for his gasoline and other travel expenses. He didn't exactly race to Seattle, though. In fact, Ed took his time getting there. "I drove my beat-up, old VW Rabbit across country for four months, crashing in hostels and in my tent, going on hiking trips in the great national parks along the way."

In early August 1996, he arrived in Seattle and rented a "little closet" for $70 a month on Seattle's Capital Hill. He was excited to be in Seattle, the hub of a lot of entertaining activities. "[It's a] great place to take off and go hike the Cascades and bike through and camp on the San Juan and British Columbia's Gulf Islands. I lived out of my backpack three days a week."

To support his outdoor passions, Ed found work as an analytical chemist. "[I] tested a lot of soils that were polluted by the Exxon Valdez disaster in Alaska." This was exciting work, but then he landed a job that he felt was the pinnacle of his working career to date. He was hired as an environmental health specialist with Seattle's Health Department.

What he enjoyed most about his job was the variety of on-site investigations he was assigned to conduct. "[I] investigated the E-coli outbreak which killed several children in the early '90s. [I ran] the department's chemical and physical hazard program, where I did cluster illness investigations on weird, unexplained illnesses. [I tested] indoor air quality, and I also [devised] one of the most comprehensive programs that dealt with the health hazards associated with illegal meth labs." It was almost a misnomer to call his occupation work because to Ed it "was a fun job."

Provincetown Campground

During the summer of 1996, before his relocation to Seattle, some of Ed's friends took time off from their dot. com lives to travel around the world. They contacted him, and he agreed to take the summer off from work and give them a guided tour of the Northeast. "[I] showed them Manhattan, Vermont, Cape Cod, and [we] camped along the way," he said. During that summer tour, Ed remembered the mosquito infested campground in Provincetown at the tip of Cape Cod—the place where Ed contracted Lyme disease.

Ed never felt well or normal again after that summer camping trip, and he couldn't understand it. He had always been a strong man—someone who biked to his job, worked out at the gym, and someone who felt he had "perfect health in the physical, mental, and spiritual sense." Now he could barely get himself out of bed to go to work, let alone bike there, and he realized that something was terribly, terribly wrong.

When Ed returned to his small, Seattle apartment in August 1996, he made an appointment with his primary care physician. At his August 9th appointment, he explained his recent, persistent symptoms to the doctor and told him that "my health was rapidly deteriorating." He asked the doctor to order a complete blood panel work-up and medication to help him sleep. Arrogantly, the doctor treated Ed like a hypochondriac and did not order the blood draw or prescribe the sleep aid medication he asked for.

After Ed mentioned the possibility that he might have

contracted Lyme disease, the doctor staunchly responded, "There is no Lyme disease in Washington State." Ed tried to reason with the doctor, explaining that he had been camping in the Northeast, a Lyme endemic area, and he hadn't felt well since then. Still, the doctor did not respond with the type of professional inquiry one would expect after hearing this kind of information. Ed realized quickly that he might as well have been talking to the wall because the doctor simply wasn't listening to his patient. Frustrated, Ed made a desperate appeal for relief, especially from his insomnia. "I pleaded with him and told him that lack of sleep was affecting my ability to drive [and] work safely on what most science professionals agree are the most dangerous, hazardous, waste sites—illegal methamphetamine labs," recalled Ed. However, the doctor did not think Ed suffered from any real disorder; and therefore, concluded his consultation without any diagnostic testing or prescribed treatment.

Ed was frustrated with the physician's quick dismissal of his request for blood testing and his concerns about Lyme disease. Unlike the doctor, Ed was certain that he was suffering from an ongoing degenerative process. Every day, he felt his illness gaining ground, and soon it began interfering with his performance on a job that posed its own life threatening dangers. The meth labs that he had investigated were sometimes filled "with booby trap bombs, explosive gases, and toxic chemicals like lead, mercury, and even radioactive materials." He had become quite skilled at investigating such sites, but lately, he was so fatigued and sleep deprived that he was not working safely. "I was walking around these sites like a zombie...,"and that was very dangerous.

Even more alarming was his failing memory. "I had a great memory, but [I] was forgetting where I parked my car three minutes ago." At first, he thought that his sleep deprivation was the probable cause for this. Fatigue had become such a problem for him at work that, at times, he had to nap in the health car for an hour in some secluded park to recoup. He was seriously concerned that if someone discovered that he was unable to work through an eight hour shift, he might lose his job. "I did whatever it took to hold on to my job, which I loved, and the health insurance that I needed to stay alive," he said.

Severe Flu

On October 29, 1996, Ed returned to see his doctor. He presented with acute symptoms resembling a severe case of the flu. "I had horrible symptoms of fevers, chills, and shortness of breath," Ed explained. Almost predictably, the physician diagnosed him with the flu. Once again, Ed questioned the doctor. "I tried to convey to my doctor that something serious was going on with my health," he said. However, the doctor did not think there was sufficient cause to suspect serious illness and would not discuss it further.

Ed went back to his doctor on November 15th, complaining of chest pains so strong that he thought he was having a panic attack or possibly even a heart attack. An EKG was performed, but it showed nothing remarkable, so the physician simply assumed that Ed was stressed out and had a panic attack. "Once again, he blew me off and treated me like a nut case," said Ed.

Ed had been told three times that there was nothing wrong with him. "I was at my wit's end," he said. He wondered if, perhaps, the doctor was right—maybe he was overextending himself. Between his job and his active, social life, he was burning the candle at both ends. Could it be that simple? Even his friends thought he was overreacting with all this talk about suffering from some sort of progressive disease. Finally, Ed was convinced that perhaps a little time away would be good for him.

Death in Paris

Ed decided to take a month off from work and travel to Paris for a little rest. "Whenever I've been at a crossroads in life, I would go to Paris and walk its streets, drink wine at cafes in the Latin Quarter on the city's left bank, take the Metro to the Pierre Lachaise cemetery [to] have a picnic on Oscar Wilde's grave, and recharge my batteries," said Ed.

Before he left for Paris, though, he saw a new doctor in Seattle—a young, Princeton educated psychiatrist, who discussed Ed's concern about possibly being ill with Lyme disease. The doctor happened to know a little about the disease since he had friends in New York who had contracted it. He told Ed that he needed to be more demanding when asking his physician for critical tests and then to get treated aggressively. Ed was very relieved to finally have met a medical professional who didn't think he was nuts. "I was so lucky to have this guy on my team," he said. With a prescription of sleeping aids in his hand, Ed left the psychiatrist's office feeling better equipped for his trip to Paris.

However, on January 4, 1997, as Ed was getting off the plane at the Charles de Gaulle airport, he felt dizzy, disoriented, and had unusual difficulties with his French. He got a taxi and found a vacancy "in an old, decrepit hotel in the Marias neighborhood of Paris on la rue Saint-Denis (the street, Saint Denis), a sketchy neighborhood of underground clubs, drug dealers, and prostitutes." The Marias was a vibrant neighborhood of mixed cultures, where the affluent and the seedy somehow learned to coexist. This was the place Ed chose as his respite, alone and isolated in a one star, run-down hotel.

By the time he was issued a key to his third floor room, he was feeling very weak and eager to collapse onto the bed. Opening the door, he dragged his backpack just inside and leaned back upon the door until it latched shut. The room was quiet and dark, yet very welcoming. His eyes were drawn to a soft street light that shone through the French doors and cast a path across the parquet flooring. He walked over to the French doors, opened them, and stepped out onto the balcony overlooking la rue Saint-Denis. The coffee terraces were empty; the book and trade shops closed. All was quiet except for some muted laughter and music coming from the restaurant-pub in the distance. In the foreground and under the shadows of one of the trees that lined the street, stood a prostitute smoking a cigarette. La rue Saint-Denis was otherwise still.

"It was perfect except I felt like I was dying and was living my own version of Thomas Mann's 'Death in Venice'—[but] in Paris," he said. Ed was very sick at this point in time. He had difficulty breathing and chills with a 103 degree fever. Sweating and dizzy, he decided to seek medical help that evening. "I staggered out onto the street and could not remember my pin number to get cash at an ATM. I could barely walk, and my knees were giving out. I was never more scared in my life, being in a foreign country and feeling like I was going to die," he recalled.

He dragged himself to a nearby pharmacy, and, in broken French, he asked the pharmacist to refer him to a doctor. "I saw a great doctor in Paris," he said, "who prescribed amoxicillin and said that I had a very strange and unusual set of symptoms unlike anything that he had seen before." Afterward, Ed returned to his hotel room where he remained isolated and sick with fever and excessive sweating. He thought he was going to die in that hotel—something like Jim Morrison—who did die in an old, fleabag hotel in Paris. Despite his fears, that didn't happen. Within two days, the amoxicillin started acting, and he began to improve.

Clueless in Seattle

After recuperating for most of January in Paris, he felt well enough to travel back to the Charles de Gaulle airport and catch a return flight to Seattle. After he arrived home, he consulted with his primary physician. He explained the health crisis he experienced in Paris, and he complained of fatigue and body aches. Despite this, Ed noticed that "[the doctor's] chart notes read 'appears well.'" *It's odd,* he thought, *that this doctor could not observe that he was suffering from some organic pathology.*

"This was my fourth appointment with [my doctor] in a period of five months. I was thinking that, at this point, my doctor would exercise some professional concern [and question] why a super healthy 31-year-old male [would] have all these weird, unexplained health episodes," Ed said. His confidence in the physician was fast waning. As an environmental health specialist with a pre-med college education and extensive work experience with unusual disorders, Ed's professional instinct told him that he was dealing with some progressive disease. "My health was going down the tubes, [yet, my doctor] dismissed me as a wack job. I trusted my doctor anyway, because I assumed that he was a professional who knew what he was doing. I tried to restrain my instinctual belief that this guy was clueless," said Ed.

Chronic Fatigue Syndrome

In late April 1997, Ed felt extreme pain in his abdomen. He hurried to the emergency room at the local hospital, and the attending doctor thought that the pain was localized in the area of his spleen. A monospot blood test was performed, and an ultrasound was taken of his spleen, but in both instances, there was nothing remarkable. He was discharged and referred to his primary physician.

At his April 28th appointment with his doctor, Ed told him that he had not felt well since his trip to Paris, four months earlier. He still felt fatigued, woozy, and experienced chills. The doctor then reviewed the test results previously performed during his emergency room admission, and said to Ed, "You have chronic fatigue syndrome (CFS)." Angered by the doctor's diagnosis, Ed told him that CFS is a "wastepaper basket diagnosis" and that he had to first rule out other diseases before coming to that conclusion. However, the doctor stood his ground and repeated his diagnosis to Ed and then concluded the visit.

Frustrated and angry at the doctor's lack of scientific methodology, Ed left the examining room and eventually consulted with his only professional ally, the "ivy league Princeton shrink." The psychiatrist was very indignant at Ed's incompetent physician and his scapegoat diagnosis. He urged Ed to go back to the medical clinic and demand a test for Lyme disease and other vector-borne infectious diseases.

Temple of Doom

By now Ed had seen his physician at the medical clinic about a half dozen times. Each time, he had been told that there was nothing wrong with him, and that he was overstressed or just imagining things. Finally, he had the boom lowered on him with a diagnosis of CFS—a totally unacceptable diagnosis from Ed's own professional perspective. With all the doom and gloom he had heard during his visits at the medical clinic, he began to refer to the clinic as "the Temple of Doom."

With renewed determination, he returned to the

infamous clinic to see his physician on May 22. He told the doctor that he was having great difficulty walking—that his knees wanted to collapse beneath him. There were times when he could barely walk. He also explained that he still had constant fatigue and chills since his trip to Paris in January. After explaining all of this, Ed told the doctor that he wanted tests performed for Lyme disease, ehrlichiosis, and babesiosis. The doctor showed immediate resistance to the idea. He told Ed, "There is no Lyme disease in Washington State." Though the physician was misinformed, Ed saw no point in arguing over statistics. Instead, he explained that he had camped throughout the Northeast just prior to presenting with symptoms and that this area certainly was endemic for Lyme disease. Then Ed told him that he would not leave the office until blood was drawn for the tests he requested.

Ed explained, "I had to take charge. This incompetent fool couldn't make a decision to save his life. I wondered if [he] even looked at my chart before my appointment. I'd brought up the Lyme disease issue several times, and he ignored it." At last, the doctor ordered the blood draw and tests that Ed wanted. About a week later, Ed called the office for the test results, and the doctor said, "You might have a little Lyme disease."

A *little* Lyme disease? Ed thought about the precious time that was wasted because the doctor had not listened seriously to his patient. "At this point, I could barely walk. [I] had fevers, chills, wooziness, and [I] thought I was going to die," recalled Ed. His doctor wanted to rerun the tests because he thought they were false positives, so he sent another blood sample to a well-known clinic in the Midwest, and the results also came back positive. Ed was then referred to an infectious disease specialist at the clinic for treatment.

Lyme Disease Treatment

Ed's first battle for truth had been fought and

finally won. He received the diagnosis that he had strongly suspected for the past year. Now, however, he faced his second formidable battle for adequate treatment of his infection. He had no idea what he was in for as he prepared to meet with the infectious disease specialist for the first time. This intelligent scientist was now a wary patient as he stood squarely on the battlefield between a rigid healthcare system on one side and practical, medical wisdom on the other.

At his June 18th appointment with the infectious disease doctor, the Lyme disease diagnosis was confirmed, and therapy was discussed. Ed advocated for a treatment of IV antibiotics since the disease was already well disseminated due to a year's delay in diagnosis. "I had central nervous disorders from the disease and Bell's Palsy," he said. The doctor did not seem receptive to the idea of IV therapy, so Ed presented him with a published medical paper on the successful use of IV antibiotic treatment for disseminated Lyme disease. The doctor laughed at the idea and said that East Coast doctors overreacted when treating Lyme disease. He had a better idea—an oral course of doxycycline—which ultimately proved to have no positive effect on Ed's health whatsoever.

From August 1997 until June 1998, Ed's health continued to deteriorate under the care of the Seattle clinic's infectious disease doctor. "I went from being a healthy person to someone who could barely get out of bed. I packed my bags and headed for New York where I saw a Lyme specialist in Manhattan. [He] referred me to Dr. Perry Orens of Great Neck, New York," Ed explained. Dr. Orens immediately started him on a prescription of IV Claforan. At that point in time, Ed had headaches so bad that he thought his head was going to explode. Then after 30 days of treatment, he began to experience convulsive-like chills and fevers every time he infused the IV antibiotics. His doctor responded by alternating his treatment between IV antibiotics and oral antibiotics over the next two years.

The Lyme War Years

Ed had learned that healing was going to be a slow journey, but he never expected to be a patient in the middle of a medical battle over treatment guidelines. Dr. Orens, who was a respected cardiologist and former teacher at Cornell University, had been treating Lyme patients with open-ended antibiotic therapies. This approach is considered by many doctors—but not the majority—as a more effective treatment for disseminated disease, albeit a blatant deviation from standard treatment guidelines. As a result, he and others like him, came under the penalizing scrutiny of the New York State Office of Professional Medical Conduct (OPMC). "[They] started cracking down on the few doctors that were treating advanced Lyme with IV antibiotics because the insurance companies did not want to pay the high cost of treatment," explained Ed.

Among them was Ed's doctor who ultimately lost his license to practice medicine, and patients lost a valuable physician with many decades of medical experience. "He was known throughout the world for his work with Lyme and other infectious diseases. He was the doctor other doctors would go to when they were sick. Dr. Orens was an example of what we should all strive to be—kind, courteous, and courageous. He saved my life," explained Ed.

This matter of threatening the medical practices of doctors treating Lyme disease with open-ended therapies came to the surface in New York State after very high profile campaigns were waged on Dr. Oren's behalf. "Letters were written and hearings were held. Dr. Orens got back his license, but he could no longer practice." As a result, physicians in that state, and in many others, have become very cautious about how they treat Lyme disease patients.

Ed personally witnessed, with disbelief, the Lyme disease war years as they were fought in New York State. He knew Dr. Orens personally, and he knew of his dedication to his patients. Ed was the last of the doctor's patients to be treated for Lyme disease prior to the revocation of his medical license. Ed felt eternally grateful to him for the treatment he had received. It gave Ed a new lease on life.

Disability and Doctors

Ed credits his New York doctor for saving his life, but that was not to say that he had fully recovered. He still had residual symptoms that made it very difficult to work. "I went on partial disability for five years, trying to hang on to my job at the health department in Seattle. I worked in horrible pain for five years. There were days when I passed out on the job from fatigue or was paralyzed by pain," Ed recalled.

Then he met a professor, who taught at the University of Washington. He agreed to see Ed as a patient in his small practice dealing with rare disorders. Every Saturday for four years, Ed consulted the doctor, who "put me back together" after a week of grueling work at the health department. According to Ed, this doctor was a "punk rocker of doctors, a political radical, who still embraced the radical politics of the 1960s without being a flaky hippie."

He practiced medicine, not because he needed the money, but because he enjoyed the challenge. "He went to India on vacation to treat lepers. He sang Clash songs while treating me. [He] was a dedicated doctor like Dr. Orens and had his license taken away by the State of Washington in February 2002." After this harsh setback, Ed did not have a treating physician to help him from week to week. His job performance plummeted, and he had to quit working altogether by June 2002.

Ed knew he had to find another doctor so that his treatment protocol would not be interrupted. He was able to locate another physician who was willing to take on his case, however, his relationship with her also ended prematurely. Within a year's time, this doctor gave a few weeks' notice and moved from Washington to practice elsewhere.

Left with enough antibiotics for only a couple of weeks, Ed was brought to despair with this information, and he feared what would happen when his medicine ran out. Acting on the tip that urgency care clinics can harbor some fine doctors, he kept his mounting anxieties at bay and worked the phones for hours. His efforts were rewarded when he found a physician who was willing to see him.

An appointment was made, and after meeting the doctor, Ed was pleasantly surprised to learn that his physician was not only knowledgeable but also empathetic and cooperative. He read through Ed's medical file, listened to him relate his medical history, and most importantly, he agreed to prescribe the medications to continue Ed's treatment protocol. He was very grateful and relieved to have found good healthcare again but was under no impression that it would last indefinitely.

The Full Life

Without a doubt, Ed's once full life changed drastically because of Lyme disease. Who wouldn't feel resentment over that? His career aspirations as an environmental health specialist came to a screeching halt. He could no longer perform the job he loved, so he stopped working. Good memories of his job still linger in his mind. "I wrote laws concerning the cleanup of meth labs. I took medical students doing their public health rounds and taught them the ins and outs of environmental health. I gave interviews to the *Seattle Times*, *National Public Radio,* and *TV News* and other televised shows from Seattle's *Northwest Afternoon* to NBC's *Today Show*."

He recalled his involvement in films like *The Graffiti Artist* with small independent writer and director, James Bolton, and other films with well known film makers like Woody Allen. "The full life of friends [and] work in the arts and sciences are gone," he said in summation. No longer will his body permit him to enjoy camping, cross country skiing, mountain hiking, or backpacking. He can't even stand long enough to serve meals to people with HIV, as he once had done. Gone, too, are the days of community activism, "fights for the creation of green space and community gardens," he reminisced.

Today, Ed lives in New York City where he continues his treatment. His physical disabilities dictate his lifestyle. He spends most of his days resting at home and exploring the more sedentary lures of the city. He is "content with reading the *New Yorker*, getting out and seeing great art, and going to the opening night of The New York Metropolitan Opera in Manhattan at Lincoln Center," he said.

It's no vacation, though. Ed continues to live with pain and fatigue. "Stress and lack of sleep cause unbearable pain, chest pain, and heart palpitations and often leads to a complete relapse. [It] also triggers shingles, another not-so-fun [disorder]," he explained. His physical pains are obvious, but his emotional pains are just as prominent. He mourns the loss of his former vivacious self, the loss of a professional and intriguing science career, and a future once filled with endless possibilities.

His father's warning that "life is short; death is long," has new meaning for him now. He's alive, yes, and grateful for all the crazy and exhilarating experiences he squeezed into the thirty-something years of his life before Lyme disease. Nonetheless, the fact remains that Ed's adventurous life had been unexpectedly shortened by chronic Lyme disease. "It can no longer compare to the life of endless possibilities that I once had," he said.

Edwin Lilley, a brilliant, scientific investigator for Seattle's Public Health Department, faced life changing circumstances in the only way he knew how—by insisting on the application of proper, scientific methodology in reaching a correct diagnosis and by following proven methods of effective treatment, even when they flew in the face of well established guidelines. Inefficient diagnostic procedures and "one size fits all" treatment guidelines were this scientist's dilemma. Overcoming those barriers to proper diagnosis and treatment consumed priceless time. Now he realizes that had he been diagnosed earlier—much earlier—and treated by a professional unfettered by rigid protocol, he might not be disabled today. He might not have had to make any professional or personal sacrifices. In fact, he might have reached a symptom-free state of health.

For Ed, that issue is water over the dam now. Lest life become even shorter and death even closer, he will carve out a new life for himself, while remaining vigilant of the latest science that might help him in his fight against chronic Lyme disease.

Seeking Help

"If you would thoroughly know anything,
teach it to others."
—Tryon Edwards

Ihave been involved with the Lyme disease community for over thirteen years. During the last eight years, I have founded and managed multiple support groups utilizing the Internet. These support websites have placed me in contact with thousands of Lyme disease patients and their loved ones from all over the world. They were all seeking the same thing—help and support in their journeys toward better health.

The experiences described in *Confronting Lyme Disease: What Patient Stories Teach Us* are relived, every day, by many in this world trying to find help for what ails them. There are definite lessons that can be gleaned from this book, and I felt they were important enough to highlight in this section for ease in finding them. The following is sound advice to follow if you believe you or a loved one may have contracted Lyme disease.

1. Get in touch with one or more Lyme disease support groups.

Support groups are often able to provide individuals with a wealth of information. There are many "real world" support groups as well as numerous support groups available over the web or via email. Support groups are often able to provide accurate information concerning Lyme disease, possible co-infections, and the names of doctors who have had success in treating the illness.

2. If you suspect Lyme disease, a proper medical evaluation for the illness and for known co-infections is needed.

Make an appointment with a doctor who has a positive record of treating Lyme disease according to the patient population. Be prepared to pay out-of-pocket expenses or travel out-of-state for an accurate evaluation and quality medical care. An experienced and knowledgeable doctor will be able and willing to explain what is happening to you, what to expect, and to answer all of your questions. The relationship you forge with the doctor will be fundamental on the road to recovery; it needs to be a positive relationship and not a source of stress or discomfort.

3. If you have Lyme disease, you will need to start treatment *immediately* and dedicate your life to getting better.

Waiting to get treatment may cause irreversible damage. Lyme disease is not a self-resolving illness. It is progressive, and immediate intervention is absolutely necessary.

4. Educate yourself, your family, and loved ones about your care.

Though it is possible to recover from Lyme disease, it may take some time, and proper support is an important component in the recovery process. Patient support is easier to give when family and friends understand what is happening to the patient. Pamphlets, books, support groups, and other resources are available to provide information about Lyme disease. There are numerous resources available on the Internet that are easy to find through any search engine. Use any, and all, resources available.

Also fundamental to recovery is a knowledgeable doctor, and yet, as key as a physician is to the healing process, he or she is only second when it comes to importance. The patient and the patient's family are the most vital people in this process. What a patient knows, understands, and communicates will be the guiding force in returning to good health.

Confronting Lyme Disease: What Patient Stories Teach Us illustrates far more than these important lessons. This book intimately portrays how Lyme disease truly affects a person—his body, mind, and soul.

Robynn Harris
Founder and Administrator of Internet Support Groups
September 2005

For More Information Contact:

Robynn Harris

Email:
Robynns_Lyme_List-owner@yahoogroups.com

Support Groups:

http://health.groups.yahoo.com/group/Robynns_Lyme_List/

http://health.groups.yahoo.com/group/Lyme-Aid/

http://health.groups.yahoo.com/group/Lyme_Aid_Parents/

http://health.groups.yahoo.com/group/Lyme_Warriors/

http://health.groups.yahoo.com/Lyme_Aid_Singles/

http://health.groups.yahoo.com/group/Oregon_Lyme

Afterword
Seeking Answers

"We learn more by looking for the answer to a question and
not finding it than
we do from learning the answer itself."
—*Lloyd Alexander*

When you are finished with this book, we would hope that you are left with a few insights. If you are simply more aware that those who are chronically ill with Lyme disease truly deserve our acknowledgment and respect for meeting extraordinary challenges, then we have accomplished something. If you are suffering from this illness or another chronic disorder, we would hope that the stories have shown that you are not alone, and that even those without a medical background are capable of learning seemingly complex information and using it to make headway in a confusing medical arena. Taking charge of your own healthcare, finding responsive medical professionals, and surrounding yourself with empathetic and helpful individuals can be key elements for sustaining hope and for overcoming the obstacles in your search for regaining health.

If, at this point, you have more questions than answers, then we have done our job. Those who shared their personal stories have given you a starting point for exploring the complexities and controversies inherent in chronic Lyme disease and for questioning specific aspects of modern medicine. We'd like to see medical consumers—that's all of us—more fully empowered with knowledge.

The willingness to dig and learn more about complex

medical matters offers an educational journey that can be fascinating and practical as well. We challenge you to seek answers for your questions, fully knowing that you will never get absolutes to all of them. We encourage you to question medical authority, and if that authority proves insufficient or counter-intuitive, listen, consider the knowledge offered, and go on to delve more deeply. When authority seems truly wise, don't accept it without thought and inquisitiveness; research on until you have reached your own conclusions. Even then, be open to modifying your stance at some point if need be.

We provide you with a very short list of resources to start you on your way. From those selected, you will be linked to additional information, such as lists of support groups or information on understanding test results. Please note from the outset, conflicting information and diversity of opinion and interpretation exist in abundance. Expect confusion, but don't let that stop you.

Caution is urged, especially when exploring the Internet. Along with medical controversy and a very sick patient population, come those who prey on the desperately ill. They may offer unsubstantiated tests or promote ineffectual or even dangerous treatments. There are also people who, while meaning well, can lead individuals down paths that may lead to harm to both health and pocketbook. While we encourage an open mind, we encourage a very sound skepticism and a large dose of common sense. Trust that you will travel far with the confidence that knowledge and critical thinking bring.

The references provided are presented for informational and educational purposes only and are not endorsed by the authors or the publisher.

Rita L. Stanley, Ph.D.
Portland, Oregon
September 2005

Reading Material

Everything You Need to Know about Lyme Disease and Other Tick-borne disorders, by Karen Vanderhoof-Forschner (Wiley & Sons, 2nd edition, 2003)

Coping with Lyme Disease, by Denise Lang with Kenneth Liegner, M.D. (Henry Hold & Company, 3rd edition, 2004)

Bull's Eye: Unraveling the Medical Mystery of Lyme Disease, by Jonathan A. Edlow, M.D. (Yale University Press, 2003)

The Widening Circle: A Lyme Disease Pioneer Tells Her Story, by Polly Murray (Saint Martin's Press, 1996)

Advice for the Patient: Drug Information in Lay Language (USP Di Vol II), (Micromedix; 24th edition, 2004)

Medical Harm: Historical, Conceptual, and Ethical Dimensions of Iatrogenic Illness, by Virginia A. Sharpe and Alan I. Faden (Cambridge University Press, 1998)

Major Organizations

Lyme Disease Foundation, Inc.
P.O. Box 332
Tolland, CT 06084-0332
http://www.lyme.org/
E-mail: lymefnd@aol.com
(860)870-0070
(800)886-LYME (5963) 24 hour information hotline

International Lyme and Associated Diseases Society
P.O. Box 341461
Bethesda, MD 20827
http://www.ilads.org
(301)263-1080

Lyme Disease Association, Inc.
5019 Megill Road
Farmington, NJ 07727
http://www.lymediseaseassociation.org/
E-mail: lymeliter@aol.com
(732)938-4834

Canadian Lyme Disease Foundation
2495 Reece Rd. Westbank
BCV4T 1N1
http://www.canlyme.com/
E-mail: jimwilson@telus.net
(250)768-0978

British Lyme Disease Foundation
P.O. Box 331
East Grinstead, West Sussex
England RH191Yt
http://www.wadhurst.demon.co.uk/lyme/
E-mail: spud@wadhurst.demon.co.uk

EuroLyme
http://health.groups.yahoo.com/group/EuroLyme/
E-mail: gilly848@ntlworld.com

Additional Resources

Centers for Disease Control and Prevention (CDC)
Home page: http://www.cdc.gov/
CDC Lyme disease: http://www.cdc.gov/ncidod/dvbid/lyme/

FDA Medical Bulletin
Lyme Disease Test Kits: Potential for Misdiagnosis
http://www.fda.gov/medbull/summer99/Lyme.html

Relapse/Persistence of Lyme Disease despite Antibiotic Therapy
12 pages of citations
http://www.lymeinfo.net/medical/LDPersist.pdf

Neuropsychiatric Lyme disease research studies at Columbia University
http://www.columbia-lyme.org/index.html

National Library of Medicine
Home page: http://www.nlm.nih.gov/

Medline Plus
A service of the U.S. National Library of Medicine & the National Institute of Health
Home page: http://medlineplus.gov/

MedlinePlus Drug Information
http://www.nlm.nih.gov/medlineplus/druginformation.html
Lyme-Borreliose-Informationen
http://www.lymenet.de/
Auf Deutsch

Infectious Disease Society of America Guidelines for Lyme Disease
http://www.journals.uchicago.edu/CID/journal/issues/v31nS1/000342/000342.html

Diagnostic Hints and Treatment Guidelines for Lyme and Other Tick-borne Illnesses
Joseph J. Burrascano, Jr., M.D.
http://www.ilads.org/burrascano_0905.html

ILADS Guidelines for the Management of Lyme Disease
http://www.tiquatac.org/ilads2003en.pdf

Listing of all Yahoo Lyme Groups
http://health.dir.groups.yahoo.com/dir/Health___Wellness/Support/Illnesses/Lyme_Disease?st=0&show_groups=1

Glossary

"Words do two major things: they provide food for the mind and create light for understanding and awareness."
—*Jim Rohn*

acidophilus – important bacteria that are naturally present in the human intestines; "friendly flora"

acute disease – an illness having a rapid onset and a short, possibly severe, course

adenomyosis – a medical condition where tissue that is normally found in the lining of the uterus is found growing within the muscular walls of that organ

ALS (amyotrophic lateral sclerosis) – also known as Lou Gehrig's disease; terminal neurological disease affecting the motor neurons and motor neuron tracts in the brain and spinal cord

analgesic – a drug that alleviates pain

anemia – lower than normal red blood cell numbers in amount of hemoglobin or in total blood volume

angina – pain or discomfort due to an inadequate flow of blood to the heart; occurs in the chest, but also may be felt in the jaw, shoulders, neck, arm, or back

antibiotic – a drug that slows or stops the growth of bacteria

antibody – an immune system protein that is made in response to an antigen such as a bacteria or virus

antigen – a substance capable of triggering an immune response in an organism

anti-inflammatory – substance that reduces fever, redness, swelling, and pain

arrhythmia – a fast, slow, or irregular heartbeat

arthropod – a member of a large group of animals that lacks a backbone and has a hard, outer skeleton (exoskeleton), a segmented body, and jointed appendages; includes insects, crustaceans, arachnids (spiders, ticks), and myriapods (millipedes, centipedes)

assay – a laboratory test or analysis

atrophy – wasting away with a loss in size of a cell, muscle, tissue, organ, or body part

autoimmune – where the immune system mistakes something naturally occurring in the organism for a foreign substance and produces antibodies to attack it

autonomic nervous system – part of the nervous system that regulates the "automatic" body functions or those not under conscious control such as sweating, heart rate, bowel functions, and blood flow

babesiosis – a malarial-like tick-borne disease; the red blood cells are infected with protozoal parasites

Babinski reflex – an abnormal reflex that can identify disease of the spinal cord and brain; when the sole of the foot is firmly stroked, the large toe moves upward and the other toes fan out; normally, the toes bunch and move downwards

bacteria – plural of bacterium

bacterium – tiny, single-celled organism, lacking chlorophyll, that usually has a cell wall, and reproduces by fission; can come in one of three forms: sphere, rod and spiral

basal ganglia – a group of four neuron clusters deep within the brain that plays a role in the control and production of movement

Bell's palsy – a disorder of the facial nerve (VII cranial) that controls the muscles of the face and results in drooping, distortion, and diminished tears; the most common type of facial paralysis

beta blocker – drug that limits the activity of epinephrine and can reduce the rate and force of the heart's pumping action

biofeedback – a method of treatment where the patient learns to control some involuntary responses such as blood pressure, heart rate, or muscle tension

blood-brain barrier – a network of tightly packed cells in the capillaries of the brain that limits the passage of many molecules into this organ

Borrelia burgdorferi (Bb) – the spirochetal (spiral-shaped) bacteria that cause Lyme disease

C. difficile (Clostridium difficile) – spore forming intestinal bacteria that, when overgrowth occurs, are the most common cause of hospital acquired diarrhea and can occur after antibiotic use; serious intestinal conditions can result from the toxins released by these organisms

candida – yeast-like fungi that normally live in the intestines but can flourish and cause disease in other parts of the body such as the mouth, genital tract, and skin when the immune system is compromised or with heavy antibiotic use

catecholamine – a chemical that acts as a neurotransmitter such as epinephrine (adrenaline), norepinephrine, and dopamine

central nervous system (CNS) – the portion of the nervous system consisting of the brain and spinal cord

cephalosporins – a family of antibiotics that are effective against specific bacteria; Rocephin, Suprax, Claforan, and Omnicef are in this group

cerebral cortex – outer layer of the cerebral hemispheres comprised of grey matter; responsible for numerous functions including consciousness, memory, speaking, voluntary activity, and sensory perception

cerebral spinal fluid (CSF) – the clear liquid that surrounds the brain and spinal cord

cervical spine – the seven bones (vertebrae) of the spine in the neck

chronic disease – illness of long-standing duration or one that comes back over and over again

chronic fatigue and immune dysfunction syndrome (CFIDS) – a disorder of unknown cause involving symptoms of persistent exhaustion that does not improve with rest and worsens with exertion; other symptoms can include neurological problems, muscle pain and weakness, and sleep disturbance

chronic fatigue syndrome (CFS) – also called chronic fatigue and immune dysfunction syndrome (CFIDS)

cognitive – relating to the ability to think, learn, remember, and reason

co-infection – infection with more than one disease-causing organism

computer axial tomography (CAT/CT scan) – a series of detailed pictures taken by x-ray to produce a cross-sectional view that is created by computer

CoQ10 (Co-enzyme Q10) – a substance found in most tissues of the body; used by the body to produce energy, protect tissues from free radical damage, strengthen the immune system, and support cardiovascular function

corticosteroid – a type of hormone produced by the adrenal glands that affects a wide range of physiologic functions and has anti-inflammatory properties; a medicine that has similar properties to the natural occurring hormone

cranial neuritis – inflammation of one or more of the 12 nerves that originate in the brain rather than the spinal cord

Creuztfeldt-Jacob disease – a very rare (about 1 per 1 million), sporadically occurring, fatal disorder of the brain hypothesized to be caused by a unique protein called a prion; more recently, new variant CJD has emerged and is commonly named "mad cow disease"

cytokine – intercellular chemical messenger proteins released by white blood cells

dementia – a mental disorder where a progressive loss of cognitive faculties results; confusion, memory, mood, personality, language, intelligence, abstract reasoning can be effected

demyelination – destruction of the myelin sheath (insulation) of certain nerves that results in loss of function of those nerves; nervous system scars or plaques can ultimately form and be visualized by MRI

disorientation – loss of or confusion about time, direction, and identity

disseminate – to spread; a disseminated infection is distributed throughout the body

dyslexia – inability or difficulty in reading that may include reversing words or letters and remembering or recognizing words

dysmenorrhea – painful menstrual periods; sometimes disabling

echocardiogram – an imaging test that uses ultrasound to examine the heart

ehrlichiosis – a tick-borne infection, similar to Rocky Mountain spotted fever; the white blood cells are invaded and infected; two types of ehrlichiosis occur in humans, human monocytic ehrlichiosis (HME) and human granulocytic ehrlichiosis (HME)

electrocardiogram (EKG) – a recording of the electrical activity of the heart

electroencephalogram (EEG) – a diagnostic test that records the electrical activity of the brain; useful to evaluate seizure disorders

electromyelogram – a test to determine whether weakness is caused by muscle disease or nerve problems; mild electric currents are used to stimulate muscle contractions, and the muscle response is analyzed

endemic county – (CDC definition for Lyme disease) one in which at least two confirmed cases have been previously acquired or in which established populations of a known tick vector are infected with Borrelia burgdorferi

enzyme – a protein that functions to increase the rate of a chemical reaction

enzyme linked immunosorbent assay (ELISA) – a laboratory test that uses an enzyme reaction to detect the presence of specific substances

epinephrine – adrenaline; a hormone that is released as a response to certain stimuli such as stress

erythema migrans (EM) rash – the early expanding rash seen in many (arguably half) cases of Lyme disease; occurs at the bite site or in distant multiple sites when the disease has disseminated; usually occurs from 2 to 30 days after the bite

etiology – the cause or origin of an illness

fibrillation – rapid, inefficient, and uncontrolled contractions of the heart muscles

fibroids – noncancerous growths in, or within, the muscles of the uterus

fibromyalgia – a chronic pain illness with widespread musculoskeletal aches, pain, and stiffness along with other symptoms such as fatigue

fifth disease – a mild childhood viral illness with flu-like symptoms and a rash; bright red cheeks are usually apparent; the name reflects that it was the fifth on a list of common childhood infections accompanied with rashes including measles, rubella, scarlet fever, and scarlatinella (variant of scarlet fever)

floaters – clumps of gel or cellular debris in the eye that can appear as spots, specks, cobwebs, spiders; can be the result of the normal aging process or can signify a serious disorder especially if they are of rapid onset

fluoroquinolones – a family of antibiotics that are effective against certain bacteria; Cipro, Levaquin, and Floxin are in this group

gastroenterologist – physician who specializes in disorders of the stomach and intestines and associated organs such as the liver and pancreas

gastrointestinal (GI) – referring to or relating to the stomach, intestines, and associated organs such as the liver and pancreas

gastroparesis – delayed emptying of the stomach due to damage to the nerves to that organ

giardiasis – a harmful protozoal infection of the gastrointestinal tract spread by contaminated water and food and direct person-to-person contact

glaucoma – an eye disease where an accumulation of fluid results in increased pressure within the eye and can lead to blindness

host – a plant or animal that harbors another organism such as a parasite; no benefit, and sometimes harm, can result to the host

hypoperfusion – diminished blood flow to a tissue or organ

IgG (immunoglobulin G) – the dominant class of antibodies and one that provides long-term protection against infection; it is produced after prolonged or repetitive exposure to an antigen

IgM (immunoglobulin M) – a class of antibodies that is formed as an initial response to an antigen

immunosuppressant – a drug or other agent capable of inhibiting or weakening the body's immune system

interstitial cystitis – a chronic bladder condition that causes pain and other problems; the bladder wall is inflamed or irritated

iritis – inflammation of the iris (colored part of the eye)

lesion – an area of body tissue altered by disease or injury

locomotor – pertaining to movement that involves progressing from one area to another

lumbar puncture – also called a spinal tap, a procedure where cerebral spinal fluid is removed from the base of the spine by needle

macrolides – a family of antibiotics that is effective against certain bacteria; Biaxin, Zithromax, Erythromycin are in this group

magnetic resonance imaging (MRI) – a diagnostic imaging technique utilizing radio-frequency waves and magnetic fields; the generated excited atoms in the study object are visualized through computer analysis

meningitis – inflammation of the lining that surrounds the brain and spinal cord (meninges) and usually caused by a bacterial or viral infection

multiple sclerosis – an illness of the central nervous system where the body's immune system attacks myelin in the brain and spinal cord

myalgias – muscle aches, pain, or tenderness

myelin – fatty substance that covers nerve cell fibers and allows for efficient conduction of nerve impulses

myoclonus – brief involuntary jerking of a muscle or group of muscles

neuroborreliosis – infection of the nervous system by Borrelia burgdorferi

neurocognitive – having to do with the ability to think and reason; includes memory, processing information, speaking, learning, concentration

neurologist – a medical doctor (M.D.) who specializes in the nervous system and its disorders

neurosurgeon – a physician who specializes in operations of the brain, nerves, and spinal cord

neutrophil – the principle microbe-eating (phagocytic) white blood cell; also releases enzymes and substances (cytokines) that affect the activity of other cells

NSAID – abbreviation for non-steroidal anti-inflammatory drug; medicine that is not a corticosteroid and used to relieve pain, swelling, and redness such as aspirin and ibuprofen

occipital lobes – the rear part of the brain (cerebral cortex) that is involved with processing information from the eyes

ophthalmologist – a medical doctor (M.D.) who specializes in the diagnosis and treatment of eye disorders

optic neuritis – inflammation of the nerve that connects the eye to the brain (optic nerve)

osteoarthritis – a degenerative condition of the cartilage of the joints – the cartilage deteriorates; the most common form of arthritis

palsy – paralysis or problems in the control of voluntary movement

Parkinson's disease – a progressive disorder of the area of the brain involved with movement; symptoms include shaking (tremor), difficulty walking, moving, and with coordination; affects about 2 of every 1,000 and usually occurs after age 50, being one of the most common neurologic disorders of the elderly

Parkinson-Plus syndrome – refers to several different neurologic diseases that initially present like Parkinson's disease, but later (a few years), different symptoms appear that allow for a more accurate diagnosis

perfusion – blood flow through a tissue or organ

peripheral nervous system (PNS) – the portion of the nervous system that lies outside of the central nervous system, including the cranial and spinal nerves

peripheral neuropathy – damage to the peripheral nerves resulting in weakness, pain, numbness, and odd sensations such as tingling or burning

peripherally inserted central catheter (PICC) – a thin flexible tube usually inserted in a vein in the arm and threaded up into the large vein just above the heart (superior vena cava); used to deliver medications, fluids, and nutrition solutions; can also be used for blood withdrawal

physiotherapist – a health care professional who treats by employing physical methods and exercise to promote healing and return to normal function

polymerase chain reaction (PCR) test – a laboratory procedure where a portion of DNA is selected and rapidly replicated to allow it to be measured

polyps – small, sack-like growths found in mucous membranes such as the rectum, uterus, bladder, and the nasal passages

protozoa (singular, protozoan)–single-celled organisms that lack cell walls and share some characteristics of animals including mobility; some can cause parasitic diseases

psychiatrist – a medical doctor (M.D.) who specializes in the treatment of mental disorders

psychogenic – of a mental or emotional origin

psychologist a professional (usually holds a Psy D. or Ph.D.) trained in the evaluation, diagnosis and treatment of mental disorders; treatment, without the use of drugs, involves counseling and/or psychotherapy

psychosis – a major mental illness that is characterized by an inability to tell the difference between the real and imaginary worlds; delusions and hallucinations occur in the disorder

psychosomatic – pertaining to physical symptoms caused or aggravated by psychological or emotional factors

radiculoneuritis – inflammation of one or more of the roots of the spinal nerves

rheumatic – relating to inflammation of joints, muscles, or tendons; pain, limitation of movement, and destruction or erosion can occur; may also refer to classify the heart problems that result from rheumatic fever (a streptococcal infection)

rheumatoid arthritis – an inflammatory disease where the immune system attacks the joints primarily but may involve other organs as well

sedimentation (sed) rate – a test to measure how quickly red blood cells settle in a test tube; can indicate inflammation or other disease processes

serology – blood test for antibodies in the blood serum (clear fluid)

single photon computed emission tomography (SPECT scan) – a diagnostic imaging technique using injected radioactive material to assess blood flow

spinal tap – a procedure where cerebral spinal fluid is removed from the base of the spine by a needle; also called lumbar puncture

spirochete – spiral-shaped bacterium

subcortical white matter – the myelin (white matter) covering the processes of the nerves under the cortex (grey matter) in the brain

syncope – a fainting spell or brief loss of consciousness

syndrome – a group of symptoms and signs that together characterize a specific condition or disorder

systemic infection – infection spread throughout the body

tachycardia – an abnormally fast heart beat

taper – to diminish gradually

thorax – the chest or rib cage: also refers to the space that contains the heart and lungs

tick-borne infection – disease transmitted by ticks

tinnitus – sensation of ringing, roaring, or buzzing sound in the head or ears

titer – measurement of the amount of a substance in a specific volume of solution (concentration)

urologist – a physician who specializes in the urinary tract of both sexes and in the male reproductive system

vasculitis – inflammation of the blood vessels; can occur in certain autoimmune disorders or with specific infections

vector – an organism, such as a tick, that can transmit disease from one host to another

vertigo – dizziness or a feeling of imbalance that has a spinning component

Western blot test – a laboratory test for specific antibodies; in Lyme disease, the specific antibodies correspond to specific areas on the Bb spirochete

About the Authors

Karen "Trish" Yerges is a prolific author with over 150 published articles on the topics of medicine, history, and art. She has extensive interviewing skills and specializes in writing narratives and biographies. Her work has appeared in newspapers and books. She has advised student writers and has received awards and recognition for her writing accomplishments. Lyme disease personally touched her life when her daughter became ill in 1999. She currently lives in northeastern Oregon with her husband and two children.

Rita Stanley, Ph.D., has done original research in the areas of physiology and biochemistry and has published in leading scientific journals such as *The Journal of Biological Chemistry, Journal of Neurochemistry,* and *Biology of Reproduction.* She was a Lyme disease support group leader for a decade at Good Samaritan Hospital in Portland, Oregon, and served on the advisory and directors' boards at the Lyme Alliance, Inc. A former Lyme patient, she lives with her husband in Portland, Oregon.

Made in the USA